MAINSTREAM ME

Clinical Haematology

MAINSTREAM MEDICINE

Clinical Haematology

D. L. BARNARD, MA, FRCP, FRCPath
*Consultant Haematologist, St James's University Hospital, Leeds
Honorary Senior Lecturer, University of Leeds*

B. A. McVERRY, MRCP, MRCPath
*Consultant Haematologist, St James's University Hospital, Leeds
Honorary Senior Lecturer, University of Leeds*

D. R. NORFOLK, MRCP, MRCPath
*Consultant Haematologist, The General Infirmary at Leeds
Honorary Lecturer, University of Leeds*

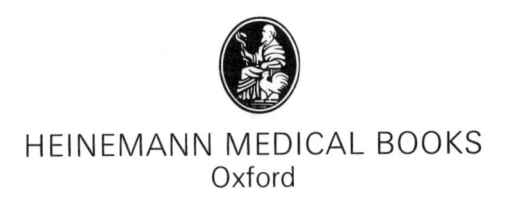

HEINEMANN MEDICAL BOOKS
Oxford

Heinemann Medical Books
An imprint of Heinemann Professional Publishing Ltd
Halley Court, Jordan Hill, Oxford OX2 8EJ

OXFORD　LONDON　SINGAPORE　NAIROBI
IBADAN　KINGSTON

First published 1989

© D. L. Barnard, B. A. McVerry and D. R. Norfolk 1989

British Library Cataloguing in Publication Data
Barnard, D. L.
　Clinical haematology.
　1. Medicine. Haematology
　I. Title　II. McVerry, B. A.　III. Norfolk, D. R.　IV. Series
　616.1'5

ISBN 0 433 00068 6

Typeset by Latimer Trend & Company Ltd, Plymouth
Printed by Biddles Ltd, Guildford and Kings Lynn

Contents

Preface vii

A PRACTICAL APPROACH TO HAEMATOLOGICAL DISORDERS

Chapter
1. Introduction 1
2. Microcytic Anaemia 10
3. Macrocytic Anaemia 23
4. Normocytic Anaemia 35
5. Haemolytic Anaemia 37
6. Haemoglobinopathies 53
7. Neutropenia 74
8. Thrombocytopenia 78
9. Pancytopenia 87
10. Leucocytosis 90
11. Thrombocytosis 97
12. Disorders of the Spleen 102
13. Bleeding Problems 110

HAEMATOLOGY TOPICS

Chapter
14. Clinical Blood Transfusion and the Use of Blood Products 127
15. Acute Leukaemia 138
16. The Chronic Leukaemias 151
17. Non-Hodgkin's Lymphomas and Hodgkin's Disease 163
18. Myeloma and the Immunocytomas 172
19. Polycythaemia 182
20. Myelodysplasia and Secondary Leukaemia 188
21. Myelofibrosis 195
22. Aplastic Anaemia 199

23.	Thrombosis	207
24.	Anticoagulant Therapy	213
25.	Liver Disease and Haematology	222
26.	Renal Disease and Haematology	228
27.	Topics in Paediatric Haematology	234
28.	Pregnancy and Haematology	247
29.	Old Age and Haematology	254
	Index	259

Preface

Haematology is an exciting and rapidly expanding subject which is at the forefront of scientific advance in many areas. Study of the haemoglobinopathies has provided the foundation for our understanding of molecular pathology and genetics in man. The relative success achieved in treating haematological neoplasms has served as a model for the treatment of malignant diseases in general. At the most practical level, a 'routine' full blood count and film report contains a wealth of information and clues which will be critically evaluated and fully understood only by an informed clinician.

This book is intended to help doctors managing patients to understand haematological processes, to arrive at a diagnosis and to deepen their knowledge of the principles of treatment. The first half of the book uses a practical approach, with emphasis on the use of salient features of the blood film report as a guide to diagnosis. The second half looks at discrete topics of primary haematological interest, at areas of general medicine with important haematological implications and at areas of growing interest.

The text is intended as an outline and guide for the general physician. Laboratory aspects, treatment schedules and the presentation of a haematological atlas are outside its scope. It should be of particular help to general physicians, and of interest to paediatric physicians, obstetricians and geriatricians.

A Practical Approach to
Haematological Disorders

Chapter One

Introduction

CONSTITUENTS OF THE BLOOD

The main cellular elements of the blood and their major functions are listed in Table 1.1. Blood cells circulate suspended in plasma whose many protein constituents include the components of the closely-interrelated coagulation, fibrinolytic and complement systems, together with antibodies present in the immunoglobulin fraction.

Table 1.1
CELLULAR CONSTITUENTS OF THE BLOOD

Cell type (synonym)	Main function
Red blood cells (erythrocytes)	Oxygen carriage (by haemoglobin)
White blood cells (leucocytes)	
(a) Granulocytes	
Neutrophil polymorphs	Phagocytosis, inflammation
Eosinophils	Host defence to certain parasites, allergy, inflammation, phagocytosis
Basophils	Allergy, inflammation, histamine release
Monocytes (macrophages in tissues)	Phagocytosis, presentation of antigens, humoral factors (e.g. interleukins, osteoclast activating factor)
(b) Lymphocytes	
B-lymphocytes	Humoral immunity (antibodies)
T-lymphocytes	Cell-mediated immunity
Platelets	Haemostasis

BLOOD CELL PRODUCTION

All the cellular constituents of the blood are derived from precursors in the bone marrow. Data from animal studies and, more recently, in vitro culture of human haemopoietic precursors demonstrate that all blood cells are derived from common pluripotential stem cells (Fig. 1.1). Under normal circumstances, the process of differentiation and maturation to the morphologically recognizable effector cells is accompanied by progressive commitment to a particular cell line.

Erythrocytes

The mature red blood cell is an anucleate biconcave disc, lacking in intracellular organelles, whose major function is the transport of oxygen bound to haemoglobin. In the process of division and maturation, red cell precursors in the bone marrow show progressive haemoglobinization accompanied by pyknosis and eventual extrusion of the nucleus. The end result is a 'reticulocyte' which is larger than the mature erythrocyte and still contains polyribosomes and occasional mitochondria. Normally, reticulocytes mature for about 24 hours in the marrow before release into

```
                    Differentiation + maturation

                                        ┌── Red cells
                                        │
                                        │┌─ Neutrophils
                                        ││
                         Committed      │└─ Monocytes/macrophages
                       ┌─ myeloid ──────┤
                       │  stem cell     ├── Eosinophils
   Common              │                │
   pluripotential ─────┤                ├── Basophils
   stem cell           │                │
                       │                └── Megakaryocytes ── Platelets
                       │
                       │
                       │  Committed     ┌── B-lymphocytes
                       └─ lymphoid ─────┤
                          stem cell     └── T-lymphocytes
```

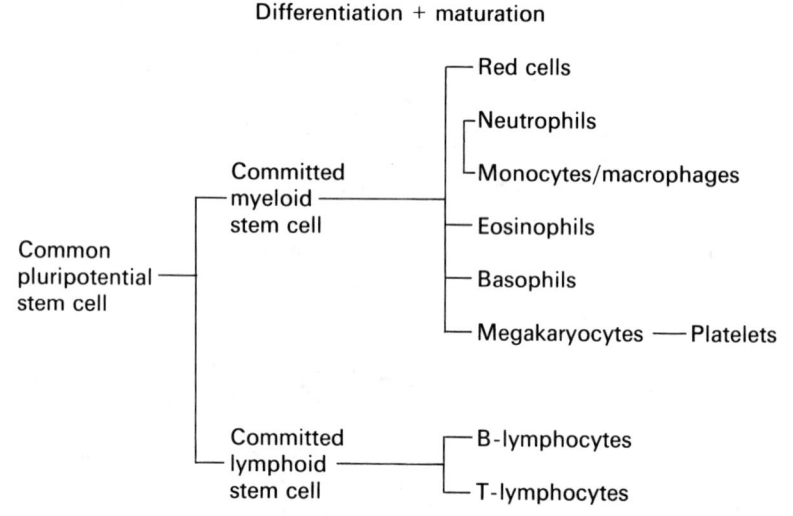

Fig. 1.1. Developmental pathway of haemopoietic cells.

the circulation and comprise less than two per cent of peripheral red blood cells. Reticulocytes may be released prematurely from the marrow in response to the increased demands of bleeding or haemolysis and their measurement is of diagnostic value. Red cells survive in the circulation for about 120 days before they are phagocytosed and digested by cells of the mononuclear phagocyte system, particularly in the spleen. Iron from haemoglobin is re-utilized, the other major breakdown product being bilirubin.

Neutrophils

After about 10 days of maturation and differentiation in the marrow, the mature neutrophil polymorph has a circulating lifespan of only a few hours. The marrow's storage pool of neutrophils is approximately 12 times that present in the blood. Whilst a venous blood sample can measure the circulating neutrophil pool, there is a further marginating neutrophil pool in close proximity to the blood vessel wall. The normal fate of neutrophils is attraction to tissue sites by inflammatory mediators or excretion in body secretions. In response to the stimulus of infection or inflammation, large numbers of neutrophils may be released into the circulating pool from the marrow and marginating pools to give the neutrophil leucocytosis characteristic of such states. Less mature forms with unsegmented nuclei may be prematurely liberated from the marrow to produce a 'left shift' in the differential white cell count.

Eosinophils

Less than one per cent of the total body eosinophils are normally present in the circulation, their normal location being the epithelial surfaces of lungs, gut and skin. Their ancestral role may have included host defence against parasitic organisms, e.g. helminths, but eosinophilia is also seen during the course of many other 'allergic reactions', including asthma and eczema.

Basophils

The characteristic granules of basophils contain histamine and heparin and are thought to have a role in the processes of allergy and inflammation.

Monocytes

Peripheral blood monocytes are in transit from marrow to tissues where they differentiate into macrophages (synonym, histiocytes). Macrophages are phagocytic cells of the mononuclear phagocyte system which often take on highly specialized roles, e.g. Kupffer cells in the liver, pulmonary alveolar macrophages and phagocytic cells in the spleen. Further vital functions of these cells include the processing and presentation of antigen to immunocompetent lymphocytes and the synthesis of many humoral factors, such as interleukins, tumour necrosis factor and osteoclast activating factor.

Platelets

Platelets are derived from the cytoplasm of megakaryocytes and fulfil an essential role in haemostasis in the form of the initial platelet plug and the provision of phospholipid membrane receptors which are important for the efficient functioning of the coagulation cascade. Megakaryocytes contain polyploid nuclei (average 16 or 32N) and there is some evidence that a high proportion of circulating platelets may be produced by megakaryocyte fragmentation in the pulmonary arterial circulation.

Lymphocytes

B-lymphocytes form a minority population (20–30 per cent) in normal peripheral blood. Their major function is antibody production in response to antigenic stimulus. T (thymus processed)-lymphocytes can be broadly categorized as providing 'help' or 'suppression' to B-cell antibody production, the normal helper:suppressor ratio being approximately 2:1. The biology of the lymphoid system is still unfolding and other recently described functions include 'natural killer cell' activity. T-lymphocytes make up 60–70 per cent of peripheral blood lymphocytes.

DEVELOPMENTAL CHANGES IN BLOOD FORMATION

The earliest site of blood formation is the yolk sac of the embryo. The liver then becomes the major site of fetal haemopoiesis until the third trimester of pregnancy. Towards term, the bone marrow gradually assumes the major haemopoietic role. At birth, red marrow occupies most of the long bones and gradually undergoes regression throughout childhood until it is confined to the axial skeleton of the normal adult. In response to increased demands, e.g. chronic haemolysis or thalassaemia major, marrow expansion with skeletal deformity may occur, and extramedullary haemopoiesis in liver and spleen may arise in patients with marrow fibrosis or malignant infiltration. The predominant haemoglobin in the fetus, haemoglobin F, is well adapted to the relatively hypoxic intra-uterine environment and is gradually replaced by adult haemoglobin A from the third trimester onwards, such that haemoglobin F concentrations form less than two per cent of total haemoglobin by the sixth month after birth.

REGULATION OF HAEMOPOIESIS

Red cell production has long been known to be regulated by the glycoprotein erythropoietin (Epo), produced by the kidneys. Epo concentrations are increased physiologically by anaemia or hypoxia and stimulate both the rate of maturation and haemoglobin synthesis of red cell precursors. Inappropriately low Epo concentrations are found in chronic renal failure and the anaemia of chronic disease (secondary anaemia). Pure Epo produced by DNA technology has recently become available and has been used therapeutically to correct the anaemia of chronic renal failure. Androgenic hormones may also stimulate erythropoiesis by increasing Epo production and sensitising erythroid precursors.

Leucocyte and platelet numbers are also held within close limits in normal health, although the precise regulatory mechanisms are less well understood. There is evidence for a hormone, thrombopoietin, which controls platelet numbers, and neutrophil release from bone marrow may be regulated by a negative feedback mechanism according to the peripheral neutrophil count. At the cellular level, the proliferation and maturation of bone marrow cells is clearly regulated by a complex interplay of positive and negative factors produced both by haemopoietic cells and cells of the supporting matrix. Recombinant granulocyte–monocyte colony stimulating factor (GM-CSF) has recently become available for clinical use, and many similar factors will be studied in the near future.

MEASUREMENT OF BLOOD CELLS

Until recent times, the only blood count parameters which could be measured with precision were the haemoglobin (Hb) concentration (colorimetric measurement of cyanmethaemoglobin) and the haematocrit (centrifugation of blood in a glass tube). Manual cell counts using counting chamber methods and estimates of cell size by microscopic techniques had a high standard error, and the 'absolute red cell indices' (Table 1.2) derived from them were of limited value in the diagnosis of anaemia. The situation has been transformed by the introduction of electronic cell counters which are able to make extremely precise measurements of cell counts and mean cell volumes (*see* Table 1.3). Mean corpuscular volume (MCV) has now become a very important diagnostic aid, and a new parameter of potential importance is the red cell distribution width (RDW), a measure of variation in red cell size (anisocy-

Table 1.2
ABSOLUTE RED CELL INDICES

Parameter	Derivation	Normal range
Mean corpuscular volume (MCV)	Hct/RCC	82–95 fl
Mean corpuscular haemoglobin (MCH)	Hb/RCC	27–32 pg
Mean corpuscular haemoglobin concentration (MCHC)	Hb/Hct	32–36 g/dl

Note: A local normal range for each parameter should be determined in every laboratory.
Hb = haemoglobin; Hct = haematocrit; RCC = red cell count.

Table 1.3
ELECTRONIC CELL COUNTERS

Direct measurements	Calculated indices
Haemoglobin (cyanmethaemoglobin)	Haematocrit (e.g. MCV × RCC)
Mean corpuscular volume (MCV)	Mean corpuscular haemoglobin (Hb/RCC)
Red cell count (RCC)	Mean corpuscular haemoglobin concentration (Hb/MCV × RCC)
White cell count (WCC)	
Platelet count	
Mean platelet volume (MPV)	

tosis). Categorization of anaemias by MCV and RDW has recently been suggested. The same parameters may be derived for platelets, although the clinical value of mean platelet volume (MPV) and 'plateletcrit' remains to be determined. It should be noted that the haematocrit is now a calculated value and does not necessarily correlate with the 'spun' packed-cell volume (PCV) which also reflects the physical rigidity of red cells and their ability to trap plasma in the red cell column. Many modern cell counters can also perform limited white cell differential counts, based on either nuclear-sizing or automated flow cytochemistry, and can be of great value in the routine laboratory by screening out those specimens which require the attention of a skilled morphologist. Automated cell counters provide no information on red cell shape changes (e.g. spherocytosis or elliptocytosis) or inclusions, and may give misleading results in the presence of red cell agglutination or rouleaux formation (spuriously raised MCV and reduced red cell count), and in vitro platelet aggregation can produce spurious thrombocytopenia.

RED CELL MORPHOLOGICAL CHANGES

Careful examination of a well-stained blood film is still the cornerstone of accurate haematological diagnosis. Table 1.4 lists some of the commonly used descriptive terms encountered in clinical practice.

Table 1.4
RED CELL MORPHOLOGY

Descriptive term	Significance
Anisocytosis	Variation in cell size
Poikilocytosis	Variation in cell shape
Microcytosis	Reduction in cell volume (e.g. iron deficiency, thalassaemia)
Macrocytosis	Increase in cell volume (e.g. megaloblastic anaemia)
Discocyte	Normal biconcave disc form
Target cell (synonym, leptocyte)	Suggests increased membrane area: volume ratio (e.g. liver disease, post-splenectomy)
Spherocyte	Small densely staining cell (e.g. hereditary spherocytosis, auto-immune haemolytic anaemia)
Elliptocyte	Lozenge-shaped cell (e.g. hereditary elliptocytosis, myelofibrosis)
Burr cell	Regular 'crimping' of cell membrane (e.g. renal failure, hypothyroid)
Acanthocyte	Irregular spiky change in membrane (e.g. liver disease)
Fragmentation	e.g. micro-angiopathic haemolysis, cardiac valve haemolysis
Sickle cell (synonym: drepanocyte)	Due to polymerization of haemoglobin S tactoids
Basophilic stippling	Dyserythropoiesis, lead poisoning
Stomatocyte	Lozenge-shaped area of central pallor (e.g. liver disease, hereditary stomatocytosis)
Red cell inclusions	
Howell–Jolly bodies	Nuclear remnants (e.g. post-splenectomy, splenic atrophy)
Heinz bodies	Denatured haemoglobin (e.g. oxidative haemolysis, unstable haemoglobin)
Pappenheimer's bodies	Cytoplasmic iron (post-splenectomy, sideroblastic anaemia)

FURTHER READING

Dacie J. V., Lewis S. M. (1984). *Practical Haematology*, 6th edn. London: Churchill Livingstone.

Hall R., Malia R. G. (1984). *Medical Laboratory Haematology*. London: Butterworths.

Chapter Two

Microcytic Anaemia

DEFINITION

The microcytic anaemias are distinguished from normocytic and macrocytic anaemias by their abnormally small red cell size, with a mean corpuscular haemoglobin (MCH) under 27 pg, or mean corpuscular volume (MCV) under 83 fl. Although the concentration of haemoglobin within the cells is usually normal, the cells are described as hypochromic because their small size makes them appear thin when spread on a blood film.

BACKGROUND

The small red cell size is a consequence of inadequate haemoglobin content and results whenever there is reduced synthesis in the developing erythroblast of haem, which contains iron, or globin (Table 2.1). Reduced haem is found when iron is low in the body (iron deficiency anaemia), or not available to the erythroblasts (despite overall stores being adequate, as in the anaemia of chronic disorders), or when there is a biochemical block in haem

Table 2.1
CAUSES OF MICROCYTIC ANAEMIA

Reduced haem synthesis
  Iron deficiency
  Iron not available (anaemia of chronic disorders)
  Synthetic pathway abnormalities (in sideroblastic anaemias)

Reduced globin chain synthesis
  α- and β-thalassaemias

synthesis (as found in the rare sideroblastic anaemias). Globin chain synthesis is abnormally slow in the thalassaemias.

IRON DEFICIENCY ANAEMIA

Aetiology

The commonest cause of iron deficiency in the West is blood loss (Table 2.2). One millilitre of packed red cells contains one milligram of iron, a huge quantity compared with any other tissue. A loss of only 500 ml (one pint) of whole blood represents the amount of iron normally absorbed from food in over 200 days.

The diet may be deficient in available iron, particularly where red meat is not eaten. Green vegetables may contain some iron in their enzymes, but fibre and phytates may impair iron absorption. In the UK, iron is added to flour, making bread a significant source. In the West, iron deficiency should not be attributed to dietary deficiency without good evidence.

Physiological states may contribute to iron deficiency (Table 2.3). There is greater than usual demand for iron in growing babies, growing adolescents (boys as well as girls), menstruation, pregnancy (where iron is needed for the increased maternal red cell mass as well as for the fetus), and lactation. It should be noted that delay in clamping the umbilical cord after delivery is very important in setting the baby up with good stores of iron, and even at one year about 70 per cent of the baby's iron is maternal in origin.

Malabsorption may present with iron deficiency anaemia, and recognition of an underlying problem like coeliac disease is vital for correct management. About 50 per cent of patients become iron deficient after a partial gastrectomy.

Table 2.2
CAUSES OF IRON DEFICIENCY

Bleeding
Increased physiological demand
Dietary deficiency
Malabsorption

Table 2.3
AVERAGE DAILY REQUIREMENT FOR IRON

Baseline requirement (e.g. for adult male)	1·0 mg
Extra requirements	
Growing adolescent	0·5 mg
Menstruation	1·0 mg
Menstruating adolescent girl	1·5 mg
Pregnancy (average overall)	2·0 mg
Late pregnancy, requirement may rise to	5·0 mg

Incidence and Geography

Iron deficiency is probably present in about 20 per cent of the world's population. It is the commonest cause of anaemia in both sexes, in all age groups and in all countries. At first sight, such a high prevalence is puzzling when iron is extremely abundant in the earth's crust (about four per cent) and when most people eat far more iron (15 mg) than they need to replace daily losses (1 mg). However, there is no method for ridding the body of excess iron, and so the body is carefully protected from the potentially harmful effects of iron excess by a sometimes too severe restriction of absorption of dietary iron. It is of interest that man evolved initially as a flesh eater and fruit and nut gatherer, and only later turned to agriculture with cereals and crops (with low iron content and absorption), which now form the world's staple diet.

In the West, iron deficiency anaemia in men is rare (0·5 per cent) and usually reflects bleeding problems, which should be fully investigated. However, nearly 20 per cent of menstruating women may be expected to increase their haemoglobin on iron therapy. Where food is predominantly rice, wheat, maize or vegetables, with little meat, iron deficiency is common. In India, for example, iron deficiency anaemia is found in over half the population, and in southern India, where Hinduism discourages meat eating, 99 per cent of pregnant women become anaemic. In Africa, where hookworm is common, and in parts of the world affected by schistosomiasis, iron deficiency from blood loss may be severe.

Symptoms and Signs

The symptoms of iron deficiency are mainly the non-specific symptoms of any chronic anaemia, with lack of energy and tiredness. In older patients, shortness of breath, exacerbation of angina, claudication or heart failure may be presenting symptoms. Iron deficiency is occasionally associated with dysphagia (Paterson–Kelly or Plummer–Vinson syndrome), which is most marked with solids. The dysphagia is caused by a postcricoid web, formed by heaped-up folds of desquamated epithelium, which can become malignant. Pica may develop in children.

The most important symptoms are those of the underlying pathology, and these are helpful in determining the likely cause of anaemia and in guiding investigations. A careful history of diet, gastro-intestinal upset, malabsorption and bleeding are important.

Details of any gastro-intestinal bleeding may suggest the site of the lesion. Haematemesis occurs when blood accumulates in the stomach or duodenum, and can result from blood swallowed from bleeding from the back of the nose. Melaena implies a blood loss of over 80 ml at a level of the caecum or higher, which allows oxidation of the blood by bacteria lower in the gut. Lesser losses are not visible (occult bleeding), but even the loss of a few millilitres daily may lead in due course to anaemia. Fresh blood passed rectally usually denotes bleeding in the colon or rectum, but it is found initially if there is heavy loss from high in the gut with rapid transit allowing no time for oxidation; melaena usually follows a little later. Fresh blood coating the outside of the stool implies a low lesion.

The signs of iron deficiency are very limited. Anaemia may be obvious. Angular stomatitis (sores at the corners of the mouth which do not heal up) is very common, but has other causes, such as poorly fitting dentures. Glossitis is usually mild, with flattened papillae, and is non-specific. Brittle nails are found in a number of patients, but the almost pathognomonic finding of koilonychia is rare and occurs only in severe long-standing iron deficiency.

Again, the signs of greatest importance are those of underlying disorders. Rectal examination should not be omitted if there is no obvious cause of iron deficiency anaemia. Careful examination of the right iliac fossa may reveal an asymptomatic caecal carcinoma.

Investigations

The depth of investigations should be determined by the clinical presentation. For a woman with anaemia and a history of menorrhagia in the UK, for example, a microcytic blood film is adequate for diagnosis and treatment. However, the subsequent response should be monitored and further investigations carried out if the response is incomplete.

In early iron deficiency, the haemoglobin may fall one or two grams from its starting level before there is a reduction below the normal range of the MCH and MCV. Soon these fall, the MCH to below 27 pg and the MCV to below 83 fl (of the two parameters, MCH is to be preferred as it can be measured more consistently throughout the country; the fall in mean corpuscular haemoglobin concentration is very late and insensitive), and the blood film becomes hypochromic with oval red cells and mild poikilocytosis.

A raised platelet count is suggestive of bleeding, but even with acute bleeding, the reticulocyte count may not be particularly raised.

When iron stores are low, serum ferritin falls below 20 µg/l, and concentrations below 10 µg/l are usual when anaemia develops. Misleadingly high concentrations are found in patients with liver inflammation. Alternative, but in general less satisfactory, measures are serum iron (low in iron deficiency, pregnancy and inflammation) and total iron binding capacity (raised in iron deficiency and pregnancy, but low in inflammation). It is common to report the ratio of these two as the percentage iron saturation, but as each is completely independently controlled, the concept is misleading.

A marrow examination is seldom needed, but may help in complicated situations. The erythroid line is increased, with late erythroblasts smaller than normal and showing delayed haemoglobinization. Iron, demonstrated by Perls' stain, is found in only a small number of erythroblasts in normal people, but it is completely absent in the erythroblasts of iron-deficient subjects. Storage iron, normally seen in the macrophages of the marrow, is utilized and disappears even before anaemia develops. If dysphagia is a problem, a lateral view of a barium swallow may demonstrate a postcricoid web.

Investigation of the underlying cause of anaemia follows normal practice but can, on occasion, be very difficult, and the vigour of pursuit should reflect the clinical context.

There are a number of problem areas. Occult gastro-intestinal bleeding may be difficult to demonstrate. Stool tests may be misleadingly negative when the bleeding is intermittent, and conversely, tests which are too sensitive pick up the normal bleeding which occurs from teeth brushing. Standard tests should detect daily blood losses of over 10 ml. Radioactive labelling of red cells, followed by stool collection, can detect losses of about 3 ml daily, but again is misleading with intermittent bleeding, and in practice this technique is seldom helpful.

There is no good and easy way to assess blood loss from menstrual periods. Heavy loss is suspected when the periods are more frequent than usual and last long (over seven days), particularly if more than the first two or three days are described as heavy. A large number of towels, inability to control loss by tampons, and large clots are again suggestive. Radioactive labelling of blood and pad collection are useful in research, and losses of more than 80 ml per period are regarded as abnormal.

Differential Diagnosis

In microcytic anaemias, ovalocytosis with pencil-shaped cells on the blood film suggest iron deficiency (see Table 2.4). In the anaemia of chronic disorders, there may be hypochromia but microcytosis is mostly mild, and the red cells are round and regular. In β-thalassaemia trait, the red cells are smaller and more numerous than in iron deficiency with a similar haemoglobin level. Formulae based on these differences are helpful to haematologists in distinguishing iron deficiency from thalassaemia, but in polycythaemia with bleeding and iron deficiency, the indices may be similar to β-thalassaemia. Target cells are prominent in thalassaemia trait, poikilocytosis minimal, and basophilic stippling may be prominent. The definitive test for β-thalassaemia trait is the haemoglobin A_2 level which is raised above 3·5 per cent. Occasionally, when severe iron deficiency complicates thalassaemia, the haemoglobin A_2 levels may be reduced below this level, but will rise again on correction of the deficiency. In the sideroblastic anaemias, a dimorphic red cell picture is usual, in which a population of affected microcytes is mixed with normal (or sometimes macrocytic) cells. Diagnosis is by marrow examination demonstrating ringed sideroblasts.

Not infrequently, patients diagnosed as having iron deficiency

Table 2.4
TYPICAL RESULTS OF INVESTIGATIONS IN MICROCYTIC ANAEMIAS

Blood features	Iron in marrow stores	Iron in erythroblasts	Serum ferritin	Serum iron	Serum TIBC	RBC HbA$_2$
Iron deficiency Oval cells usual	↓	↓	↓	↓	↑	N
Inflammatory anaemia Normocytic or mild microcytosis	↑	↓	↑	↓	↓	N
Sideroblastic anaemia Dysplastic and dimorphic	↑	Rings	↑	↑	N	N
β-thalassaemia trait Marked microcytosis RBC count near normal Low RDW	N	N	N	N	N	↑

HbA$_2$ = haemoglobin A$_2$; N = normal; RBC = red blood cell; RDW = red cell distribution width; TIBC = total iron binding capacity

fail to respond to iron therapy. This is usually because they are not taking the iron medication (the stools should be a dull black if they are complying), but sometimes the bleeding is too fast for iron replacement to keep up, and this is particularly so where the underlying disorder cannot be treated, e.g. hereditary telangiectasia. Rarely, malabsorption or concurrent infection limits the response to oral iron therapy. Sometimes the diagnosis of iron deficiency is wrong, most often where β- or α-thalassaemia trait have been overlooked.

Complications

Anaemia itself can give rise to complications such as cardiac failure. Iron deficiency could, in theory, cause widespread problems, as it is an essential element in vital enzymes such as the cytochromes. In theory also, iron deficiency can reduce immunity to infection, but in practice there is little evidence that these possibilities have any clinical implications. Indeed, community surveys have shown surprisingly few harmful effects, even in people with quite severe anaemia, compared with those with normal blood counts, although recently there has been evidence that iron deficiency can lead to dementia and poor thermal regulation in the elderly.

Treatment

Prevention of iron deficiency anaemia worldwide is largely a matter of diet and control of parasitic infections. In the West, flour for making bread may be supplemented with iron. Individual prophylactic iron therapy is not recommended in vegetarians unless iron deficiency has become a problem. In pregnancy, it is usual to give iron and folate supplements if the diet is known to be poor; otherwise, the haemoglobin level is monitored throughout pregnancy with a view to investigation and appropriate treatment if it falls below about 11·0 g/dl. It should be remembered that patients who develop high haemoglobin levels because they do not expand their plasma volume in the normal way in pregnancy are more vulnerable to pre-eclamptic toxaemia (*see* Chapter 28).

Treatment of iron deficiency anaemia is directed towards iron replacement and correction of the underlying cause. Oral therapy is straightforward in most patients. Ferrous sulphate 200 mg (63 mg iron) three times daily is cheap and effective. It should improve the haemoglobin level by about one gram per week until it is normal. The blood film in a patient responding to iron treatment is dimorphic, showing a new population of normal cells mixed with the hypochromic cells made when the patient was still iron deficient. A few patients are troubled by minor nausea, abdominal pains or changed bowel habit, and these side-effects are usually overcome by reducing the dose (fewer tablets daily or tablets with less iron, such as ferrous fumarate), or taking the tablets after meals (which also reduces the amount of iron absorbed). In children, a liquid preparation such as ferrous fumarate in syrup with 45 mg iron per 5 ml (or in diabetics a sugar-free preparation such as iron edetate) is useful. Iron is normally continued for about two or three months after correction of the anaemia, with the intention of building up body stores.

Some patients are unable to take oral iron. This is common in the vomiting of early pregnancy, and in Crohn's disease where the iron can irritate the gut. In these situations, iron can be given intramuscularly (by deep zigzag injections to avoid unsightly skin discoloration) or intravenously. Use of the latter route has been complicated by anaphylactic reactions, and so infusion of the dose needed to correct total body iron should be started very slowly with more careful observation over the first 20 minutes. Blood transfusion, with all its risks, is seldom justified in treating chronic iron deficiency.

THE ANAEMIA OF CHRONIC DISORDERS

This term is applied to an anaemia found in chronic inflammatory disorders, which include chronic infections (e.g. tuberculosis or wound infections), collagen diseases and some malignancies (particularly Hodgkin's disease). The anaemia is usually normocytic, but there may be hypochromia, and sometimes microcytosis. The disorder is extremely common, but often misdiagnosed.

The salient abnormality, known as reticulo-endothelial blockade, is that iron is not released normally from the macrophages in the marrow or at sites of local inflammation, such as the joints in rheumatoid arthritis, where a great excess of iron may be found. Leakage from these cells results in high serum ferritin concentrations, which help distinguish this disorder from iron deficiency. Serum iron, which normally comes predominantly from macrophage release, is reduced, and the erythroblasts in the marrow are deprived of iron, mimicking genuine iron deficiency.

Iron therapy is not helpful. Correction of the anaemia depends on treatment of the inflammation, e.g. by antibiotics for tuberculosis, or disease-modifying agents in rheumatoid arthritis. The block in iron release is thus corrected, and the red cells return to normal.

SIDEROBLASTIC ANAEMIAS

Definition

In these rare disorders of erythropoiesis, a ring of iron-containing granules is seen around the nuclei of some erythroid precursors (ring sideroblasts). Impaired haem synthesis leads to iron accumulation in the mitochondria, which lie close to the erythroblast nucleus.

Classification and Aetiology

Hereditary sideroblastic anaemia is rare and is usually transmitted as a sex-linked recessive disorder, with males presenting with moderate anaemia between infancy and early adulthood. Acquired forms of sideroblastic anaemia are more common (*see* Table 2.5).

Pathology

A variety of biochemical defects in haem synthesis have been described, but often a more general abnormality causing dyserythropoiesis (abnormal red cell production) and anaemia is found.

Symptoms and Signs

The symptoms and signs are those of a chronic anaemia, and of any underlying disease. Mild splenomegaly is usual in the

Table 2.5
CAUSES OF SIDEROBLASTIC ANAEMIA

Congenital
  Sex-linked, with males affected clinically
  Mother may show occasional microcytes in blood and rings in marrow

Acquired
  Primary or idiopathic
                              Common in people over 60 years old
  Secondary
                              Drugs, e.g. isoniazid, pyrazinamide
                              Toxins, e.g. alcohol, lead
                              Haematological diseases, e.g.
                                Folate or vitamin B_{12} deficiency
                                Myeloid leukaemias
                                Myelodysplasia
                              Collagen diseases
                              Carcinomas
                              Uraemia

congenital variety, but uncommon otherwise except when sideroblastic change complicates myelodysplasia (*see* Chapter 20).

Investigations

In the hereditary form, anaemia with marked microcytosis is found and the blood film shows a dimorphic pattern with a population of microcytic cells mixed with normal cells. Although a microcytic population of cells is also found, as expected, in the acquired variety, the majority of red cells may in fact be dysplastic and macrocytic with a raised MCH.

Marrow examination is essential to demonstrate the ringed sideroblasts, and usually shows the increased iron stores expected in dyserythropoietic anaemias. Serum ferritin may be high, and serum iron raised.

Differential Diagnosis

The blood film may be mistaken for iron deficiency, but the dimorphic and dysplastic red cells should suggest sideroblastic change. Mixed deficiencies of iron and folate may produce a similar dimorphic picture, but in addition may show right shift, pancytopenia or circulating megaloblasts.

Complications

In the congenital variety of sideroblastic anaemia, haemochromatosis with pigmented skin, diabetes and liver disease may occur from increased iron absorption, even though transfusion is seldom needed. With acquired sideroblastic anaemia, repeated transfusions are often required and these increase the chances of developing haemochromatosis. The idiopathic variety may be a clonal disease, and may be complicated by myelodysplasia and acute leukaemia (*see* Chapters 15 and 20).

Treatment

If drugs or chemicals causing a sideroblastic process can be stopped, the problem is reversible. Where anaemia is clinically troublesome, treatment with folic acid (5 mg daily) has sometimes proved beneficial even when no formal deficiency can be demonstrated. Oral pyridoxine (200 mg daily for adults) improves the anaemia in a small proportion of patients with sideroblastic anaemia; treatment should be continued for at least three months as the response may be slow.

Severe anaemia will require regular transfusion with packed cells and if possible, the blood should be processed in some manner to reduce leucocytes (to lessen the likelihood of subsequent febrile transfusion reactions from cytotoxic antibodies – *see* Chapter 14). In young patients with a good prognosis, iron chelation therapy to prevent iron overload should be considered.

Prognosis

The prognosis reflects the underlying diseases and the development of any complications.

THE THALASSAEMIAS AND MICROCYTOSIS

The thalassaemias are discussed in detail in Chapter 6. The decreased globin synthesis leads to a microcytic anaemia, and some of the thalassaemias may be mistakenly diagnosed as iron deficiency. Iron therapy should be avoided unless coexisting iron deficiency has been established.

Beta-Thalassaemia

In β-thalassaemia trait, there is usually a mild and asymptomatic microcytic anaemia, with haemoglobin levels usually above 9 g/dl, but these levels may fall, especially in pregnancy. Diagnosis is suspected, particularly in patients from appropriate countries, from the marked microcytosis in relation to the haemoglobin level (e.g. MCH 20 pg or MCV 60 fl with haemoglobin 10 g/dl), from the minimal anisocytosis (reflected in the low red cell distribution width) and plentiful target cells. It is confirmed by finding a haemoglobin A_2 level greater than 3·5 per cent. Serum ferritin is normal, unless there is concurrent iron deficiency, when the haemoglobin A_2 levels will be lower than expected.

Alpha-Thalassaemias

Where three of the four genes are affected (haemoglobin H disease), a moderate microcytic anaemia is usual, with haemoglobin levels of 7 to 10 g/dl. The red cell indices are similar to β-thalassaemia, but the haemoglobin A_2 levels are normal. Haemoglobin H levels of about 10 per cent are found, and plentiful precipitates from free β-chains can be shown as inclusions in the red cells by staining with vital stains such as cresyl blue.

Where two genes are affected (α-thalassaemia trait), there is usually no clinical problem but the blood shows a microcytic anaemia with normal iron studies and normal haemoglobin A_2 levels. Confirmation is often difficult and may require repeated and prolonged examinations for the occasional red cells showing precipitated globin by vital stains. Chain synthesis rates or DNA analysis may be needed for diagnosis.

FURTHER READING

Bothwell T. H., Charlton R. W., Cook J. D., Finch C. A. (1979). *Iron Metabolism in Man*. Oxford: Blackwell Scientific Publications.

Jacobs A., ed. (1982). Disorders of iron metabolism. *Clinics in Haematology*, **2**(2).

Chapter Three

Macrocytic Anaemia

DEFINITION

Macrocytosis of red cells is usually defined by a mean corpuscular volume (MCV) greater than 95 fl. Although the presence of macrocytosis often suggests abnormal red cell production in the marrow, it may also occur as a physiological phenomenon (e.g. in the neonate and in pregnancy) or be an artefact of automated cell sizing (Table 3.1).

Table 3.1
CAUSES OF MACROCYTOSIS

Physiological	*Haematological disease*	*Miscellaneous*	*Spurious artefactual*
Normal neonate	Megaloblastic anaemia	Alcohol toxicity	Rouleaux
Pregnancy	Myelodysplasia (primary or secondary)	Hypothyroidism	Cold agglutination
	Reticulocytosis (bleeding or haemorrhage)	Drugs (e.g. anticonvulsants, oral contraceptives)	
	Aplastic anaemia	Chronic hypoxia	
	Leuco-erythroblastosis		
	Congenital dyserythropoietic anaemias		

DIFFERENTIAL DIAGNOSIS

A full history and clinical examination, together with examination of a well-stained blood film, will normally lead to a presumptive diagnosis which can be confirmed by further tests, such as bone marrow biopsy and vitamin assays. In modern practice, the presence of moderate uniform macrocytosis in the absence of anaemia will strongly suggest excessive alcohol ingestion. Myelodysplasia should be suspected in the elderly patient or the recipient of previous cytotoxic chemotherapy and will normally be accompanied by characteristic changes in white cell or platelet morphology (*see* Chapter 20). Reticulocytes have a higher MCV than mature erythrocytes and, in the anaemic patient, an increased reticulocyte count will suggest active bleeding or haemolysis. Patients with aplastic anaemia or leuco-erythroblastosis (due to bone marrow infiltration) often show moderate macrocytosis. Bone marrow aspiration and biopsy should be performed wherever possible to avoid misdiagnosis, the particular problem being myelodysplasia in the elderly patient.

MEGALOBLASTIC ANAEMIAS

'Megaloblastosis' describes characteristic morphological changes in the marrow due to impaired DNA synthesis. Deficiencies of vitamin B_{12} or folic acid are by far the most common causes of megaloblastosis in clinical practice, but any interference with DNA synthesis may produce similar changes in blood and marrow (Table 3.2). Red cell precursors retain immature nuclei in fully haemoglobinized cells (nuclear–cytoplasmic asynchrony), and many red cells die before release into the circulation (ineffective erythropoiesis). Changes are also seen in the granulocyte and megakaryocyte series with typical 'giant metamyelocytes' and increased nuclear segmentation, respectively. In the peripheral blood, oval macrocytic red cells are seen, together with hypersegmented neutrophil polymorphs (five or more lobes to the nucleus). The MCV tends to rise with increasing severity of anaemia to around 130 fl, but may fall to normal in advanced cases as large numbers of small red cell fragments are formed. Advanced cases may also have leucopenia and thrombocytopenia and may occasionally be complicated by spontaneous bleeding. Ineffective haemopoiesis is reflected in raised levels of plasma unconjugated

Table 3.2
CAUSES OF MEGALOBLASTOSIS

Folic acid deficiency
Vitamin B_{12} deficiency
Drug induced:
  Folate antagonists (e.g. methotrexate)
  DNA-synthesis inhibitors (e.g. hydroxyurea, mercaptopurine)

Haematological malignancy:
  Erythroleukaemia
  Myelodysplasia

Metabolic:
  Rare abnormalities of folate or vitamin B_{12} metabolism
  Orotic aciduria

---

bilirubin and lactate dehydrogenase. Folate is an essential co-enzyme in the synthesis of thymidylate (a pyrimidine constituent of DNA), whereas vitamin B_{12} catalyses the demethylation of circulating tetrahydrofolate to the precursor of active folate polyglutamates (Fig. 3.1). Deficiencies or abnormal metabolism of either vitamin B_{12} or folate leads to a reduced rate of DNA synthesis whilst RNA synthesis is unimpaired.

FOLIC ACID DEFICIENCY

Folates (usually in the form of reduced polyglutamates) are present in a wide variety of foods with particularly high levels in liver, green vegetables and yeasts. Up to 90 per cent of folate content may be destroyed if food is overcooked (particularly by boiling). The normal daily requirement for folate is around 100 μg and the average body store (mainly in the liver) of 10 mg provides only about four months' reserve. Dietary folate is absorbed with high efficiency, the major site being the proximal jejunum. The causes of folate deficiency can be classified as dietary, failure of absorption or increased utilization or losses (Table 3.3). Dietary folate deficiency is the most common of these causes. Folate requirements are relatively higher in infancy, and deficiency is predisposed by recurrent infection, feeding difficulties and inappropriate diet (e.g. the fashionable goat's milk is a

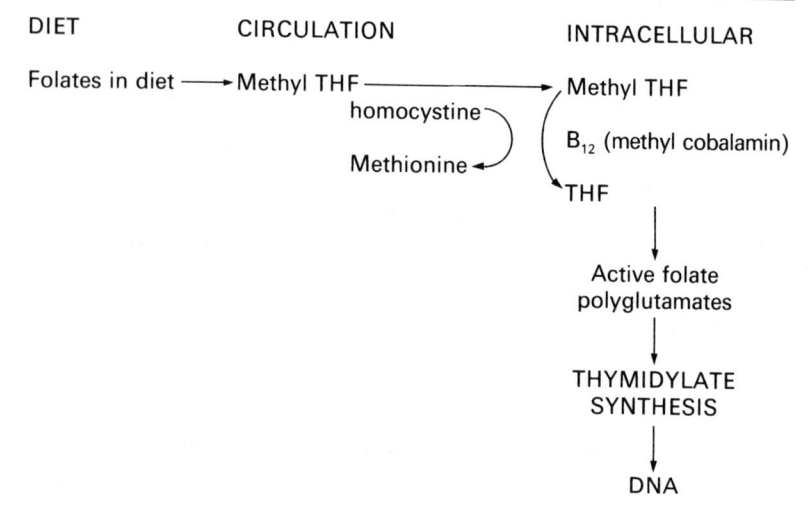

```
DIET              CIRCULATION              INTRACELLULAR
Folates in diet ──▶ Methyl THF ────────────▶ Methyl THF
                         homocystine ⎫
                                      ⎬      B₁₂ (methyl cobalamin)
                         Methionine ⎭
                                              ↓
                                              THF
                                              ↓
                                         Active folate
                                         polyglutamates
                                              ↓
                                         THYMIDYLATE
                                          SYNTHESIS
                                              ↓
                                             DNA
```

Fig. 3.1. Inter-relation of vitamin B_{12} and folate in DNA synthesis (THF= tetrahydrofolate).

very poor source of folate). In later life, dietary folate deficiency is usually seen in the context of poverty, old age, alcoholism and poor dietary education and culinary techniques. Several factors often coexist in the same patient, and other nutritional deficiencies, such as vitamin C, may also be present.

In view of the marginal folate balance of the normal diet and the limited body stores, folate deficiency is a sensitive indicator of malabsorption states such as gluten enteropathy. Certain drugs, particularly anticonvulsants and the contraceptive pill, have been implicated in folate malabsorption, although the precise mechanism is uncertain. Increased folate requirements are a feature of chronic haemolytic anaemias, including thalassaemia major and sickle-cell disease. Megaloblastic anaemia is a particular problem in primary myelofibrosis and may contribute to the pancytopenia. The ineffective haemopoiesis of the myelodysplastic syndromes may also be complicated by folate deficiency. A combination of increased demands and reduced dietary intake probably accounts for the increased incidence of folate deficiency in many patients with malignant or chronic inflammatory diseases (e.g. tuberculosis, Crohn's disease and rheumatoid disease). As folate is not highly protein-bound, excessive losses may occur in haemo- or peritoneal dialysis and precipitate negative folate balance where dietary intake is also poor.

Table 3.3
CAUSES OF FOLATE DEFICIENCY

Dietary:	Common at extremes of life (*Note*: low folate content of goat's milk, 'tea and cake' diet of elderly) Poor nutritional education/overcooking/fad diets/protein-calorie malnutrition/poverty
Malabsorption:	Gluten enteropathy (coeliac disease) Dermatitis herpetiformis Tropical sprue Crohn's disease Jejunal resection Amyloid Lymphoma (rare) Whipple's disease
Increased utilization/losses:	Haemolysis (increased Myeloproliferative disorders marrow Myelodysplasia/leukaemia activity) Malignant and chronic inflammatory diseases (often in combination with poor diet) Severe psoriasis/exfoliative dermatitis Congestive heart failure—increased urinary losses Haemodialysis Pregnancy (especially multiple) Prematurity (increased surface area to weight ratio)
Drug-related:	Antifolate drugs (e.g. methotrexate) Anticonvulsants (e.g. phenytoin) Oral contraceptives

Clinical Features

The clinical picture will largely reflect the context in which folate deficiency occurs. In infancy and childhood, folate deficiency will cause failure to thrive and may be associated with impaired growth. The insidious onset of anaemia may lead to presentation with angina pectoris or heart failure in the older patient. Conversely, the diagnosis may be made on a routine blood count in the presymptomatic stage. Common clinical features include angular stomatitis, glossitis and mild jaundice (raised unconjugated bilirubin). Megaloblastic change can occur in all actively dividing cells, especially the epithelial lining of the gut, urinary and genital tracts. Reduced fertility is common in severe megaloblastic anaemia and recent, but as yet unconfirmed, evidence suggests that the incidence of spina bifida and other neural tube defects may be reduced by preconceptual folate supplements. Neurological complications are clearly less common in folate than in vitamin B_{12} deficiency (see below), but well-documented cases have been described.

Diagnosis

The blood and marrow changes are indistinguishable in folate or vitamin B_{12} deficiency (see below). A therapeutic trial of pharmacological doses (100 µg daily) of folate will produce a haematological response, but higher doses will also produce a response in vitamin B_{12} deficiency with the risk of precipitating subacute combined degeneration of the cord. In current practice, it is usual to measure the serum and red cell folate levels. The more convenient radioassays have now largely replaced microbiological assays (e.g. *Lactobacillus casei*). Serum folate concentrations are sensitive to recent dietary changes, and red cell folate levels may give a better picture of body folate stores. However, red cell folate measurement may be confounded by recent transfusion or a high reticulocyte count (false normal), or by severe vitamin B_{12} deficiency in which levels are reduced (inability to produce intracellular polyglutamates). The increased urinary excretion of formimino glutamic acid (Figlu test) in folate deficiency is unreliable and non-specific and has been replaced by the specific assays. Correction of the in vitro deoxyuridine suppression test by folate but not B_{12} is occasionally used for final confirmation.

VITAMIN B_{12} DEFICIENCY

The cobalt-containing vitamin B_{12} molecule is largely present in the body in the deoxyadenosyl form, although methyl cobalamin is the active co-enzyme in the folate pathway (Fig. 3.1). In nature, vitamin B_{12} is exclusively synthesized by micro-organisms, and the only dietary source for humans is food of animal origin, particularly liver and kidney (although vegetables and fruits contaminated by bacteria can be a minor source). The vitamin is stable to cooking temperatures. The normal daily requirement to replace losses in faeces and urine is around 1–2 μg, the average Western diet contains up to 30 μg per day and normal body stores are of the order of 1–3 mg (i.e. up to four years' reserve).

Vitamin B_{12} absorption occurs by a highly efficient active process centred on the terminal ileum. Gastric acid and enzymes in the upper gastro-intestinal juices release free vitamin B_{12} which forms a one to one molecular complex with gastric intrinsic factor (IF) produced by the parietal cells of the body of the stomach. The stable IF–B_{12} complex actively attaches to receptors on the mucosa of the terminal ileum and B_{12} is transported to the portal bloodstream. Dietary vitamin B_{12} may also attach to non-IF R-binder proteins in gastric juice from which they are normally released by pancreatic enzymes such as trypsin. In the circulation, vitamin B_{12} is largely bound to the glycoprotein transcobalamin I (TCI), although the 10 per cent or so of B_{12} available for use as a co-enzyme is attached to TCII.

Vitamin B_{12} deficiency is virtually always due to impaired absorption, although dietary deficiency is occasionally seen in strict vegetarians (vegans). The causes of vitamin B_{12} deficiency are listed in Table 3.4. Vitamin B_{12} deficiency is inevitable after total gastrectomy and lifelong replacement therapy should start postoperatively. Dietary deficiency also occurs in up to 15 per cent of patients after partial gastrectomy, often in association with iron deficiency. Blind-loop syndromes are due to the growth of colonic bacteria in the upper ileum, often after surgical anastomoses or inflammatory bowel disease. Such patients often have high concentrations of serum folate. Extensive surgical resection of the terminal ileum (usually for Crohn's disease) may also result in megaloblastic anaemia. Chronic vitamin B_{12} malabsorption is common in tropical sprue; conversely, clinically significant vitamin B_{12} deficiency is very rare in adult coeliac disease. Significant vitamin B_{12} deficiency is similarly uncommon in atrophic gastritis and chronic pancreatitis. Heavy infestations of the ileum by the fish tapeworm (*Diphyllobothrium latum*) is a rare cause of B_{12} deficiency in regions of raw fish ingestion (e.g.

Table 3.4
CAUSES OF VITAMIN B_{12} DEFICIENCY

Dietary:
  Strict vegans (but uncommon even in this group)

Impaired absorption:
  Intrinsic factor deficiency—Addisonian pernicious anaemia
  —Gastrectomy

  Ileal abnormalities—Often associated with megaloblastic anaemia
  　　Surgical resection (usually for Crohn's disease)
  　　Stagnant loop syndromes—postsurgical or jejunal diverticulosis
  　　Crohn's disease
  　　Tropical sprue
  　　Fish tapeworms
  　　Congenital defects of vitamin B_{12} absorption

  　—Rarely associated with megaloblastic anaemia
  　　Coeliac disease
  　　Chronic pancreatitis
  　　Atrophic gastritis
  　　Zollinger–Ellison syndrome

Abnormal B_{12} metabolism:
  Congenital TCII deficiency
  Methyl malonic aciduria
  Inactivation of B_{12} by nitrous oxide or cyanide

Drug-related:
  e.g. metformin

Scandinavia, Japan and North America). A variety of drugs, including metformin, phenytoin and alcohol, may reduce vitamin B_{12} absorption and cause decreased serum concentrations, but the histamine H_2-receptor antagonists cimetidine and ranitidine, which block acid production by gastric parietal cells, do not appear to cause IF deficiency. Rare cases of congenital deficiency of the vitamin B_{12} carrier protein TCII have been reported (normal total serum B_{12} levels but megaloblastosis and neurological problems), and long-term exposure to nitrous oxide may cause megaloblastosis and neuropathy (especially in the intensive care unit) due to oxidation of methyl cobalamin.

Addisonian Pernicious Anaemia (PA)

This is the commonest cause of vitamin B_{12} deficiency in northern European populations (incidence about 120 per 100 000). There is a relative female preponderance, and an increased incidence of PA and other auto-immune diseases (e.g. auto-immune thyroid disease, diabetes mellitus and Addison's disease) in family members. The peak age of onset is 60 years. Patients with PA have a virtually unmeasurable output of gastric IF, reduced secretion of pepsin and hydrochloric acid, and high concentrations of serum gastrin. There is gastric mucosal atrophy, frequently with an inflammatory infiltrate and intestinal metaplasia. Males appear to have a higher than standard incidence of gastric carcinoma.

Evidence for an auto-immune aetiology of PA includes the presence of detectable IF antibodies in the serum of more than 50 per cent of patients and in the gastric juice of more than 80 per cent. Antibodies may be 'blocking' (preventing the formation of IF–B_{12} complexes) or 'binding' (inhibiting the binding of the complexes to ileal receptors). Gastric parietal cell antibodies are much less specific for the diagnosis of PA, being found in up to 20 per cent of normal elderly women and in many other auto-immune diseases. Further evidence of an auto-immune basis is the ability of corticosteroid therapy to improve B_{12} malabsorption in some patients.

Clinical Features

The general symptoms of anaemia, stomatitis and glossitis are indistinguishable from severe folate deficiency. Marked anorexia is common and the combination of anorexia, weight loss, anaemia and jaundice often raises the clinical suspicion of gastric or colonic neoplasia. In severe cases with leucopenia and thrombocytopenia, infection and bleeding may occur. The classical neurological syndrome of vitamin B_{12} deficiency is 'subacute combined degeneration of the cord'. Patients complain of ataxia, paraesthesia, weakness and occasional mental disturbance. Visual disturbance due to optic neuritis may occur. There is usually evidence of peripheral neuropathy and demyelinating lesions in both the posterior and lateral columns of the spinal cord. Lhermitte's sign is often positive. It has been suggested that impaired production of s-adenosyl methionine, an essential component of myelin, is the basis for this syndrome. Neurological complications occasionally precede the development of anaemia.

Diagnosis

As with folate deficiency, a therapeutic trial of physiological doses of parenteral vitamin B_{12} may be performed. However, this rather time-consuming process has now largely been replaced by specific measurement of serum vitamin B_{12} concentrations. Microbiological assays (e.g. *Lactobacillus leishmanii*) remain the 'gold standard' but have largely been replaced in routine use by the more convenient radio-isotope dilution assays. Many radioassays give higher results than the microbiological tests (possibly owing to the use of relatively non-specific R-binder proteins in the assay rather than IF), and a single normal B_{12} measurement should not deter further investigation if a strong clinical suspicion of vitamin B_{12} deficiency remains. Correction of the deoxyuridine suppression test by vitamin B_{12} but not by folate may be a useful confirmatory measure. Measurement of increased urinary methyl malonic acid excretion may also be useful in doubtful cases (deoxyadenosyl cobalamin is an essential co-enzyme for the conversion of methyl malonic acid to succinyl CoA).

Once a diagnosis of vitamin B_{12} deficiency has been made, further tests may be employed to determine the cause. A full clinical history should include details of previous surgery, drugs and abnormal diet, and often leads to a presumptive diagnosis. Tests for IF antibodies are becoming increasingly available, and it is usual to screen for other common auto-antibodies. Measurements of gastric acid and IF output are now rarely performed. Vitamin B_{12} absorption tests remain of value in confirming and localizing the site of B_{12} malabsorption. The classical procedure is the Schilling test in which the patient ingests a small dose (1–2 µg) of radiolabelled vitamin B_{12} orally after a loading dose of parenteral vitamin B_{12} to saturate binding proteins. Urinary excretion of radioactive vitamin B_{12} is then observed over 24 hours (normally 10 per cent or more of the ingested dose is excreted). If malabsorption is confirmed by a reduced urinary excretion, the test is repeated using B_{12} bound to IF which corrects the deficit in classical PA. Use of two isotopes of cobalt (e.g. ^{57}Co, ^{58}Co) allows both parts of the test to be carried out simultaneously for convenience, although less precise results may be obtained.

The test may also be confused by malabsorption due to megaloblastic change in the small intestinal mucosa, and it is recommended that the B_{12} absorption tests are carried out as a confirmatory measure only after several weeks of treatment have been given.

TREATMENT OF MEGALOBLASTIC ANAEMIA

Patients presenting with severe anaemia (haemoglobin concentrations of only 2 or 3 g/dl are occasionally seen) should be started on treatment with both vitamin B_{12} and folic acid until the results of specific assays are available. Transfusion should be avoided unless absolutely necessary in view of the real danger of precipitating cardiac failure, often with a fatal outcome. If transfusion is unavoidable, one or two units of concentrated red cells should be given slowly, under diuretic cover and with removal of a similar volume from the other arm. In the absence of a definitive diagnosis, folic acid should never be given alone to patients with megaloblastosis because there is a risk of initiating severe neurological symptoms in patients with vitamin B_{12} deficiency. Marrow recovery with treatment may occasionally be accompanied by severe hypokalaemia, and it is common practice to prescribe potassium supplements.

Folate deficiency can virtually always be treated orally with pharmacological doses of folic acid (5 mg daily) even in patients with coeliac disease and malabsorption. The underlying cause of deficiency must be identified and corrected wherever possible. Long-term folic acid supplements may be necessary in patients with chronic haemolytic anaemias. Prophylactic folic acid (about 400 µg per day) is commonly given in pregnancy, although the trend is to reserve it for patients in high-risk socio-economic groups. Folate supplements are routinely given to premature infants and patients on chronic haemodialysis.

Relatively few causes of vitamin B_{12} deficiency are amenable to correction, e.g. dietary advice or surgical correction of blind loops. Most patients will require intramuscular injections of vitamin B_{12}, hydroxocobalamin now being preferred to cyanocobalamin because of the higher tissue retention. It is conventional to give five or six daily doses of 1000 µg of vitamin B_{12}, after which body levels are satisfactorily maintained by a three-monthly schedule. There is no evidence that larger or more frequent doses have any advantage.

Evidence of a haematological response to folic acid or vitamin B_{12} is seen in a reticulocyte count rising from about the third day of treatment and peaking at about day seven. Red cell precursors in the marrow become normoblastic within 48–72 hours and a rise of haemoglobin of the order of 1 g/dl per week is seen. Suboptimal or ill-sustained response should lead to the exclusion of concomitant iron deficiency (or consumption of iron stores by the marrow response). White cell and platelet counts normalize in 7–14 days, but the response of neurological symptoms may be very slow and often incomplete.

FURTHER READING

Chanarin I. (1979). *The Megaloblastic Anaemias*, 2nd edn. Oxford: Blackwell Scientific Publications.

Hoffbrand A. V., ed. (1976). Megaloblastic anaemia. *Clinics in Haematology*, 5(3), 471–769.

Chapter Four

Normocytic Anaemias

This is the commonest type of anaemia encountered in practice and is characterized by normal mean corpuscular volume and mean corpuscular haemoglobin levels. Unlike hypochromic microcytic and macrocytic anaemias, it does not suggest a working diagnosis or a specific line of investigation to follow. While this form of anaemia may be secondary to bleeding or haemolysis, it is very commonly associated with the 'anaemia of chronic disease', i.e. anaemia related to an infectious, inflammatory or neoplastic disease.

A particularly useful test in this situation is the reticulocyte count. A normal physiological response to anaemia is hyperplasia of erythropoiesis in the marrow with early release of reticulocytes into the circulation. Therefore, the absence of a reticulocytosis in the presence of anaemia suggests impaired bone marrow function. The blood film report may suggest the presence of a reticulocytosis by demonstrating increased polychromasia.

Anaemia with an appropriately raised reticulocyte count suggests the presence of:

1. haemorrhage
2. haemolysis
3. a partially treated anaemia secondary to a haematinic deficiency such as iron, folic acid or vitamin B_{12}.

When a normochromic, normocytic anaemia is not associated with an appropriate reticulocyte response, the differential diagnosis is multiple (Table 4.1).

The anaemia of chronic disease is a common cause of a normochromic, normocytic anaemia. The cause of anaemia in this disorder is multifactorial and includes disturbed iron metabolism, reduced erythropoiesis in the bone marrow and reduced

Table 4.1
CAUSES OF A NORMOCHROMIC, NORMOCYTIC ANAEMIA

Anaemia of chronic disease
Primary bone marrow dysfunction, e.g. leukaemia, myelodysplasia
Bone marrow damage secondary to drugs, radiation or infiltration
Renal disease
Reduced function of the pituitary, thyroid or adrenal glands

red cell survival. The presence of normal or increased iron stores in the marrow with reduced quantities in normoblasts suggests a block in the transfer of iron to these cells. Clinically, it presents as a moderately severe anaemia (haemoglobin 9–11 g/dl). Serum iron and transferrin saturation levels may be very low, but serum ferritin concentrations are normal, excluding a diagnosis of iron deficiency. The anaemia of chronic disease is a diagnosis of exclusion. Most patients do not require treatment, nor has any form of treatment, apart from blood transfusions, been shown to be helpful, unless of course the underlying cause can be corrected, e.g. the control of rheumatoid arthritis by disease modifying agents. Unlike the anaemia of renal failure, it is not known if these patients would respond to erythropoietin. However, there is some evidence that this is unlikely, as in experimental situations, such anaemias are associated with a degree of erythropoietin resistance.

FURTHER READING

Williams W.J., Beutler E., Ersler A.J., Lichtman M. A., eds. (1986). *Haematology*. New York: McGraw-Hill.

Chapter Five

Haemolytic Anaemia

DEFINITION

The circulating red cell, lacking a nucleus, is unable to synthesize protein for growth and repair. Normal survival (mean 120 days) depends upon the maintenance of the membrane, cytoplasm and haemoglobin in the correct state to provide adequate flexibility to traverse the circulation, and to maintain the primary function of oxygen exchange between lungs and tissues. The absence of intracellular organelles leads to reliance on the anaerobic glycolytic pathway (Embden–Meyerhof pathway) to provide the energy necessary for these active processes. Reducing power (critical to preserve the integrity of the lipid membrane and haemoglobin) is provided both by the glycolytic and pentose phosphate pathways. Many inherited and acquired abnormalities or insults to these processes will lead to shortened red cell survival. Haemolytic anaemia occurs when red cell losses exceed the capacity of the marrow to compensate.

CLASSIFICATION OF HAEMOLYTIC ANAEMIAS

It is convenient to classify haemolytic anaemias as either inherited or acquired, and as 'intrinsic' (due to abnormalities of the red cell itself) or 'extrinsic' (due to external insults) (Table 5.1).

GENERAL CLINICAL AND LABORATORY FEATURES OF HAEMOLYSIS

Destruction of red cells in excess of marrow production leads to anaemia and variable jaundice. Chronic haemolysis may also be

Table 5.1
CLASSIFICATION OF HAEMOLYTIC ANAEMIAS

Inherited
  (i) *Intrinsic*

Membrane abnormalities	Hereditary spherocytosis
	Hereditary elliptocytosis
Enzyme abnormalities	Glycolytic pathway (energy and reducing power)
	Pentose phosphate pathway (reducing power)
Haemoglobin disorders	Thalassaemias
	Abnormal haemoglobins

  (ii) *Extrinsic*

Abnormal environment	Abetalipoproteinaemia

Acquired
  (i) *Intrinsic*

Dyserythropoiesis	Paroxysmal nocturnal haemoglobinuria
	Myelodysplasia
	Dyserythropoietic anaemias

  (ii) *Extrinsic*

Auto-immune haemolysis	Warm antibody
	Idiopathic
	Secondary (e.g. systemic lupus erythematosus, lymphoma)
	Drug-induced
	Cold antibody
	Cold haemagglutinin disease
	Secondary to infection
	Paroxysmal cold haemoglobinuria
Allo-immune haemolysis	Post-transfusion
	Haemolytic disease of the newborn
Drug-induced haemolysis	Auto-immune
	Hapten
	'Innocent bystander'

Environmental problems	Micro-angiopathy
	Thrombotic thrombocytopenic purpura
	Haemolytic uraemic syndrome
	Cardiac haemolysis
	March haemoglobinuria
	Hypersplenism
	Liver disease
	Renal disease
	Toxins
	Thermal injury

complicated by pigment gallstone formation. Splenomegaly, due to hypertrophy of reticulo-endothelial cells in the spleen, is present in many forms of haemolytic anaemia. The classical peripheral blood feature of haemolysis is an increase in the reticulocyte count, as red cell precursors are prematurely released from the marrow. In severe cases, nucleated red cells may also be seen in the peripheral circulation. The larger size of the reticulocytes is manifest as a moderate elevation of mean corpuscular volume (MCV) on the electronic cell counter. Specific red cell changes, such as spherocytosis or cytoplasmic inclusions, may help in differential diagnosis. The bone marrow typically shows erythroid hyperplasia, and expansion of the marrow cavity may lead to skeletal deformity characteristic of such chronic diseases as untreated β-thalassaemia major.

Haem from the destroyed red cells is catabolized to bilirubin which is converted in the liver to a water soluble diglucoronide before excretion (Fig. 5.1). In haemolytic anaemias, the jaundice reflects increased levels of unconjugated ('indirect') bilirubin which circulates bound to albumin. Unconjugated bilirubin does not enter the urine, hence the term 'acholuric jaundice', but urobilinogen, produced from the bacterial breakdown of bilirubin entering the gut, is readily detected in the urine.

Haptoglobins in plasma bind free haemoglobin formed during haemolysis, and the complex is removed by the mononuclear–phagocyte system. Consequently, low or absent plasma haptoglobin levels are a feature of chronic haemolysis. When red cells are destroyed in the circulation ('intravascular haemolysis'), free haemoglobin may be detected in plasma and urine if the rate of

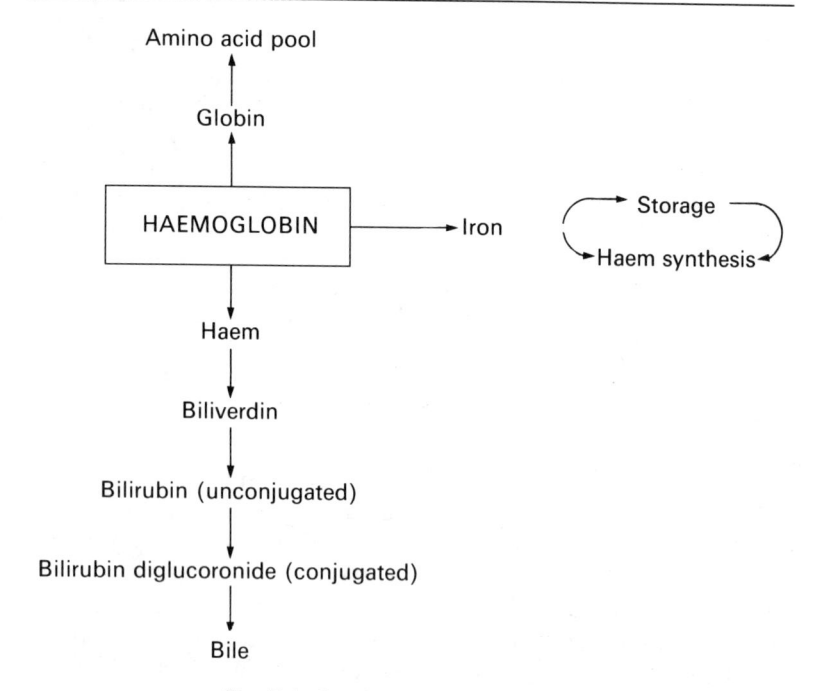

```
           Amino acid pool
                  ↑
               Globin
                  ↑
         ┌─────────────────┐                    ┌──→ Storage ──┐
         │   HAEMOGLOBIN   │────→ Iron          ⟨              ⟩
         └─────────────────┘                    └→ Haem synthesis ←┘
                  ↓
                Haem
                  ↓
              Biliverdin
                  ↓
        Bilirubin (unconjugated)
                  ↓
   Bilirubin diglucoronide (conjugated)
                  ↓
                 Bile
```

Fig. 5.1. Catabolism of haemoglobin.

production exceeds the binding capacity of the haptoglobins. In such states, the pigment methaemalbumin is formed and may be detected by spectroscopy or Schumm's test. In chronic intravascular haemolysis, haemoglobin is degraded to haemosiderin in renal tubular cells and may be detected by iron staining of centrifuged urine deposits.

COMPLICATIONS OF CHRONIC HAEMOLYTIC ANAEMIA

Pigment gallstones may occur in any chronic haemolytic anaemia, and leg ulceration may be a feature of certain congenital forms (e.g. sickle-cell disease and hereditary spherocytosis). Increased red cell turnover readily leads to folate deficiency and may limit the capacity of the marrow to compensate. 'Aplastic crises' have long been recognized in congenital haemolytic anaemias in which there is a temporary loss of red cell production lasting two or three days. In the face of shortened red cell survival, this results in a rapid fall in haemoglobin concentration with absence of circulating reticulocytes. This occasionally fatal complication is now known to be caused, in most instances, by the human parvovirus (B19), the agent of erythema infectiosum ('fifth disease') which may also cause hydrops foetalis and stillbirth if infection is acquired in utero.

INHERITED HAEMOLYTIC ANAEMIAS

Membrane Abnormalities

Hereditary spherocytosis (HS)

This is the commonest inherited haemolytic anaemia in Northern Europeans and is usually transmitted in an autosomal dominant fashion. Most patients are heterozygotes, as the homozygous form is probably lethal. It is a heterogeneous disorder, and a number of red cell membrane defects—particularly of the membrane cytoskeletal protein, spectrin—have now been identified in different families. The degree of anaemia is highly variable and most patients demonstrate mild jaundice and splenomegaly. Patients with the more severe variants may present with prolonged neonatal jaundice, although exchange transfusion is only rarely required. Pigment gallstones early in life are common and leg ulceration may occur. The blood film shows the characteristic microspherocytes which are produced by the removal of membrane by phagocytic cells as the red cells traverse the spleen. The electronic cell counter commonly displays a raised mean corpuscular haemoglobin concentration (MCHC). Spherocytosis may be a feature of any state where red cell membrane loss occurs (Table 5.2). The red cells of HS show a reduced ability to withstand osmotic stress, a phenomenon utilized in the 'osmotic fragility test' where the degree of red cell lysis is determined in different concentrations of saline and compared with normal control cells.

Patients with mild, compensated haemolysis may not need specific treatment although it is wise to prescribe folate supplements and undertake regular clinical review to avoid the complications of cholelithiasis and skeletal deformity. Splenectomy produces near normalization of red cell lifespan in most patients

Table 5.2
MAJOR CAUSES OF SPHEROCYTOSIS ON THE BLOOD FILM

Hereditary spherocytosis
'Warm antibody' haemolytic anaemias
ABO haemolytic disease of the newborn
Clostridium welchii septicaemia
Post-splenectomy (small numbers)

but results in a lifelong susceptibility to infection by encapsulated bacteria, particularly pneumococcus. The operation is avoided in early childhood if possible as the infection risk is clearly higher in children. Relative indications for splenectomy include persistent hyperbilirubinaemia, poorly compensated haemolysis, cholelithiasis, aplastic crises and leg ulceration.

Hereditary elliptocytosis (HE)

This is another autosomal, dominantly inherited disorder produced by a variety of red cell membrane abnormalities. The characteristic red cell is rod-shaped or oval, and the number of abnormal cells varies considerably from case to case. Most patients have no evidence of increased haemolysis, the spleen is rarely enlarged and osmotic fragility is normal or minimally increased. The minority of cases with significant haemolytic anaemia usually respond well to splenectomy. The rare homozygous individual may present a bizarre red cell picture with fragmented cells and spherocytes. Similar abnormal morphological features may be seen in the neonate with heterozygous HE, often leading to diagnostic confusion. Examination of the parents' blood films usually reveals the diagnosis, and the infant's red cells assume the classical appearance between three and six months of age.

Enzyme Abnormalities

Glycolytic pathway

In this metabolic pathway, glucose is converted to pyruvate with the generation of energy in the form of ATP and reducing power as NADH.

Pyruvate kinase deficiency, albeit rare, is the commonest inherited abnormality of this pathway and produces an autosomal recessive non-spherocytic haemolytic anaemia. Haemolysis is extravascular, as effete red cells are removed in the reticuloendothelial system. Presentation is with anaemia and jaundice, usually early in life. Moderate splenomegaly is common and haemoglobin levels range from 5–10 g/dl. Symptoms of anaemia may be surprisingly mild as there is a compensatory reduction in the oxygen affinity of haemoglobin (due to raised concentrations of 2,3-diphosphoglycerate). The blood film shows a considerable increase in reticulocytes and characteristic 'prickle cells' may be seen. Enzyme activity is now usually measured directly in the routine laboratory but enzyme variants may be missed if kinetic studies are not performed, usually the remit of the specialized laboratory. Patients should receive folate supplements, and transfusion is necessary in a significant minority. Splenectomy is beneficial to some extent in most patients and should certainly be considered in those requiring regular transfusion. Other inherited enzyme deficiencies of this pathway are very rare; they produce a similar haematological picture and some are associated with neuromuscular abnormalities or mental retardation.

Failure of reducing power

Glucose-6-phosphate dehydrogenase (G6PD) is an essential enzyme in the pentose–phosphate pathway (hexose–monophosphate shunt) which produces reducing power in the form of NADPH. The genes for G6PD are carried on the X-chromosome; therefore, inheritance of abnormal isoenzymes is sex-linked. The common (normal activity) isoenzymes are type A in black (African origin) populations and type B in Caucasians. Abnormal variants are common in many populations and seem to have arisen by natural selection in malarial areas, where they may afford relative protection against falciparum malaria. Reduced G6PD concentrations or activity leads to the oxidation and denaturation of haemoglobin and subsequent red cell membrane rigidity under conditions of oxidative stress. The type A variant in Negroes is associated with acute haemolysis after the ingestion of many drugs, for example antimalarials, sulphonamides and phenacetin (Table 5.3). Haemoglobinuria, anaemia and jaundice occur 72 hours after ingestion and are self-limiting, as reticulocytes with higher G6PD levels enter the blood. Patients with the

Table 5.3
SOME DRUGS WHICH MAY CAUSE HAEMOLYSIS IN GLUCOSE-6-PHOSPHATE
DEHYDROGENASE (G6PD) DEFICIENCY

Phenacetin
Sulphonamides (including sulphasalazine)
Nitrofurans (e.g. nitrofurantoin)
Chloramphenicol (Mediterranean-type G6PD deficiency)
Antituberculosis agents (streptomycin, para-aminosalicylic acid, isoniazid)
Antimalarials (primaquine, mepacrine, chloroquine; quinine is safe in Negroes)
Naphthalene (mothballs)
Methylene blue

Mediterranean variant of G6PD may develop sudden severe intravascular haemolysis after exposure to broad beans (favism). Haemolysis may also occur after oxidative drugs or infections. G6PD deficiency may also produce prolonged neonatal jaundice, and kernicterus may occur.

The blood film between haemolytic episodes is normal in G6PD deficiency. Contracted or fragmented red cells are seen during crises, and Heinz bodies (denatured haemoglobin) may be seen by supravital staining. Many screening tests of varying sensitivity are available, but levels may be normal in the presence of increased reticulocytes. More sophisticated assays, electrophoretic and kinetic studies may be needed for final diagnosis.

Haemoglobin Disorders

Reduced red cell survival is present in the homozygous form of many pathological haemoglobin variants and the thalassaemia syndromes. Haemoglobinopathies and thalassaemia are covered in detail in Chapter 6. Patients with sickle-cell disease have markedly reduced red cell survival, as irreversibly sickled cells are trapped in the microvasculature and reticulo-endothelial system. Attempted marrow compensation results in a reticulocyte count of 10–15 per cent in most patients, and skeletal deformity due to expansion of the marrow cavity is sometimes seen. Haemolytic crises may occur in which a dramatic, occasionally life-threatening, fall in haemoglobin is accompanied by a rise in reticulocyte count.

Red cell survival is also significantly reduced in patients doubly heterozygous for haemoglobins S and C (haemoglobin SC disease). Such patients run haemoglobin levels of the order of 10–12 g/dl (compared with 6–8 g/dl in sickle-cell disease), largely due to the higher oxygen affinity of the SC variant. Patients homozygous for haemoglobin C (mainly Negroes of West African origin) have a chronic mild haemolytic anaemia associated with mild splenomegaly and many target cells on the blood film. Homozygosity for haemoglobin E (mainly seen in South East Asia) also produces a mild chronic haemolytic anaemia although the co-inheritance of haemoglobin E and β-thalassaemia trait results in a very severe haemolytic diathesis.

Most patients with structural haemoglobin variants producing methaemoglobinaemia (haemoglobin Ms) or altered oxygen affinity (e.g. haemoglobin Chesapeake) have minimal or absent haemolysis and are usually suspected because of an otherwise unexplained cyanosis (haemoglobin Ms), anaemia (low affinity haemoglobins) or polycythaemia (high affinity haemoglobins).

The unstable haemoglobin variants result from mutations affecting the stable tertiary structure of haemoglobin. Globin chains precipitate in the red cell where they may be detected, in splenectomized individuals, as Heinz bodies by supravital staining ('congenital Heinz-body haemolytic anaemias'). A large number of such haemoglobin variants have now been described, including haemoglobins Koln, Hammersmith and Bristol. Patients have a chronic, non-spherocytic haemolytic anaemia of variable severity, which is made worse by oxidant drugs and which may be helped by splenectomy. Investigations include haemoglobin electrophoresis and demonstration of haemoglobin precipitation on heating.

The basic pathological process in thalassaemia syndromes is the unbalanced rate of production of α- and non α-globin chains. Excess α-globin chains in β-thalassaemia, and vice versa in α-thalassaemia, lead to the formation of insoluble inclusions and red cell membrane damage. The relative failure of haem production results in excessive iron incorporation into the red cells. Patients with thalassaemia major syndromes have grossly ineffective erythropoiesis; most red cells die within the marrow cavity and the features of marrow cavity expansion and extramedullary haemopoiesis in liver and spleen dominate the clinical picture (*see* Chapter 6).

Abetalipoproteinaemia

In this inherited disorder of lipid metabolism, there is abnormal incorporation of lipids into the red cell membrane resulting in characteristic 'acanthocytosis' of red cells and mildly reduced red cell survival.

ACQUIRED HAEMOLYTIC ANAEMIAS

Dyserythropoiesis

Abnormal red cell production in the bone marrow from many causes leads to reduced red cell survival. Ineffective erythropoiesis is a feature both of megaloblastic anaemias (vitamin B_{12} or folate deficiency) and of the primary myelodysplastic syndromes (*see* Chapter 20). Rare syndromes of congenital dyserythropoietic anaemia have also been described, diagnosis depending on the typical morphological features of blood and bone marrow, exclusion of other predisposing diseases, and examination of family members.

Paroxysmal nocturnal haemoglobinuria (PNH) is an acquired red cell abnormality characterized by the presence of a clone of red cells with abnormal sensitivity to membrane lysis by complement. That the underlying disorder arises in a myeloid stem cell is shown by similar abnormalities demonstrable in granulocytes and platelets. The PNH clone may appear de novo or arise in an abnormal marrow (especially in aplastic anaemia or myelodysplastic syndromes). Conversely, patients with PNH may later develop aplastic anaemia or, less commonly, acute myeloid leukaemia. Clinically, the classical presentation is with anaemia and the passage of dark urine containing haemoglobin (i.e. intravascular haemolysis). Haemosiderin is detected in the urinary sediment even between bouts of clinical haemolysis (a useful screening test), and the definitive diagnosis is made by demonstrating lysis of the patient's red cells in vitro in the presence of activated complement. In the classical Ham's test, complement in the patient's serum is activated by acidification ('acid lysis test').

Complications of PNH include a tendency to thrombosis in unusual sites, including the hepatic veins (Budd–Chiari syndrome) and cerebral veins. Severe intermittent abdominal pain, chronic renal failure and susceptibility to infection may occur. Treatment with steroids may be useful if haemolysis is severe or other complications supervene, and many patients need iron supplements to replace that lost in the chronic haemoglobinuria. Transfusion must be with red cells washed free of plasma, otherwise very severe haemolysis may be precipitated. The prognosis of PNH is highly variable. Spontaneous remissions may occur, but up to 50 per cent of patients are dead within 10 years. Diagnosis is not infrequently made after many years of symptoms.

Auto-immune Haemolytic Anaemia (AIHA)

The antibodies causing red cell membrane damage in the auto-immune haemolytic anaemias are broadly classified by the temperature at which their activity is greatest. 'Warm' antibodies show maximum activity at body temperature (37 °C) and are most commonly of the IgG subclass. IgG antibodies are often 'incomplete' (*see* Chapter 14) and are best detected by the direct antiglobulin (Coombs') test (DAT). Haemolysis due to warm antibodies is usually extravascular, antibody-coated red cells being removed in the reticulo-endothelial system. 'Cold' antibodies are maximally active below body temperature and normally produce clinical problems only under unusual environmental conditions. They are usually of the IgM subclass and may produce intravascular haemolysis by the activation of complement on the red cell membrane with rupture of the erythrocyte.

Warm antibody AIHA

This is commonly idiopathic but is seen with increased frequency in patients with other auto-immune diseases, especially systemic lupus erythematosus (SLE). An increased frequency of AIHA is also seen in chronic lymphocytic leukaemia, non-Hodgkin's lymphoma and Hodgkin's disease, and may be seen after virus infections in childhood. Certain drugs, classically methyldopa, may initiate AIHA.

The onset of AIHA may be rapid or insidious. On occasions, a rapid fall in haemoglobin may have fatal consequences. Mild splenomegaly and jaundice are usual, and features of an underlying disorder (e.g. lymphoma or SLE) may be present. The blood count often shows mild macrocytosis, reflecting the raised reticulocyte count, and spherocytes, polychromasia and nucleated red blood cells may be seen in the blood film. The direct Coombs' test (DAT) is usually positive and bone marrow examination shows erythroid hyperplasia. The level of haemoglobin will depend on the relative rates of red cell production and destruction.

Corticosteroids are the primary treatment for AIHA. The main immediate effect is to impair the ability of macrophages in the reticulo-endothelial system to recognize and phagocytose the antibody-coated red cells. In the longer term, steroids will reduce antibody production and may have an effect on any underlying disease. Most patients respond within 2–3 weeks of treatment, but some may require dangerously high maintenance doses of steroids to prevent recurrence. Alternative or adjunctive treatments include splenectomy and the use of cytotoxic or immunosuppressive agents, such as cyclophosphamide and azathioprine.

Cold antibody AIHA

Cold antibody AIHA may be acute or chronic and related to a variety of underlying disorders (Table 5.4).

Table 5.4
COLD ANTIBODY HAEMOLYTIC ANAEMIA

Type	Antibody specificity
Cold haemagglutinin disease (CHAD)	I
Due to infection	
Mycoplasma pneumoniae	I
Infectious mononucleosis	I or i
Secondary to	
Lymphomas	i
Carcinomas	I

Note: I antigen predominates on adult red cells and i on fetal erythrocytes.

Cold haemagglutinin disease (CHAD)

CHAD is associated with the presence of an indolent and often clinically inapparent low grade non-Hodgkin's lymphoma in which the abnormal clone of cells produces an IgM antibody capable of agglutinating red cells in the cold. Patients are usually elderly and present with painful acrocyanosis of the extremities on exposure to cold. In severe cases, the ingestion of cold food or liquids may be painful. The antibody may occasionally retain activity at body temperature ('high thermal amplitude') and cause a chronic intravascular haemolytic anaemia. Examination of the blood film shows agglutination of red cells which may produce a falsely raised MCV on the electronic cell counter. A monoclonal immunoglobulin (always of IgM kappa specificity) corresponding to the cold antibody activity may be detected in the serum.

In milder cases of CHAD, the avoidance of cold and the protection of extremities by mittens, ear-muffs etc., may be highly beneficial. In the more severe cases, the use of alkylating agents such as chlorambucil may slowly reduce the cold agglutinin titre, but long-term administration increases the risk of secondary leukaemia. Steroids are rarely beneficial. Relief of acute symptoms may be achieved by plasma exchange which efficiently lowers the cold agglutinin level (IgM is predominantly intravascular in distribution).

Secondary cold agglutinin disease

This condition is most commonly related to infection, classically by *Mycoplasma pneumoniae*, but also with various virus infections including infectious mononucleosis and cytomegalovirus. Depending on the characteristics of the antibody induced, haemolysis may occur about two weeks after infection but is usually mild and transitory.

Paroxysmal cold haemoglobinuria (PCH)

PCH was originally described in patients with syphilis who experienced bouts of haemoglobinuria on exposure to cold. In modern practice, PCH is generally idiopathic or secondary to viral infection. The characteristic Donath–Landsteiner antibody is a cold-reactive IgG antibody which recognizes the P blood group antigen. Treatment with corticosteroids is usually successful (syphilis must, of course, be treated with penicillin).

Allo-immune Haemolytic Anaemia

Transfusion of red cells possessing antigens that are lacking in the recipient may lead to immunization. On subsequent transfusion, red cells of the offending group may lead to a secondary immune response and a 'delayed transfusion reaction' (*see* Chapter 14).

Allo-immunization of rhesus(D)-negative women during pregnancy or by transfusion may cause the formation of IgG 'immune' antibodies capable of crossing the placenta and producing haemolytic disease of the newborn in subsequent rhesus(D)-positive infants.

Drug-induced immune Haemolytic Anaemia

Drugs may cause immune haemolysis by three main mechanisms (Table 5.5). Certain drugs (classically methyldopa) appear to modify antigens on normal red cells and induce the formation of auto-antibodies. The direct Coombs' test (DAT) is positive in up to 10 per cent of individuals on methyldopa, but overt haemolysis is much less common (less than one per cent).

Other drugs react with red cell membranes, and antibodies may be produced to the drug/membrane complex (hapten formation). Examples of this type include treatment with large doses of penicillins or cephalosporins. The DAT is usually positive.

The third major mechanism is the so-called 'innocent bystander' phenomenon, whereby the interaction of drug (often loosely associated with the red cell) and antibody causes complement activation and lysis of the red cell membrane. Examples

Table 5.5
DRUG-INDUCED HAEMOLYSIS

Auto-immune	*Hapten*	*'Innocent bystander'*
Methyldopa	Penicillins	Quinidine
L-dopa (rarely)	Cephalosporins (in high dosage)	Sulphonamides
		Chlorpropamide

include quinidine and sulphonamides. Detection of antibodies in the patient's serum may depend on the presence of the drug.

Severe drug-induced AIHA is usually responsive to steroids and drug withdrawal. A positive DAT alone is not an indication to stop methyldopa. Hapten and innocent bystander type haemolysis usually stop when the drug is eliminated from the circulation.

Micro Angiopathic Haemolysis

This is characterized by the presence of fragmented red cells (schistocytes) in the blood film. Haemolysis due to traumatic fragmentation of red blood cells may be seen in patients with prosthetic heart valves, especially if leakage or regurgitation is present. This problem was much more common with the older ball and cage type of valve (e.g. Starr valve) but may also be seen with the more modern xenografts. The characteristic blood picture is accompanied by jaundice and haemosiderinuria (a sensitive indicator of chronic intravascular haemolysis). Bedrest, control of heart failure and careful transfusion may reduce the severity of haemolysis, but valve replacement is often the only permanent solution if the anaemia is severe. A similar blood picture is seen in the syndrome of march haemoglobinuria where red cell damage is caused by prolonged running or other repetitive trauma.

Red cell fragmentation in small blood vessels, due to the presence of fibrin strands acting in the manner of 'cheese-wires', is typically seen in disseminated intravascular coagulation and disorders such as haemolytic uraemic syndrome, thrombotic thrombocytopenic purpura, malignant hypertension and pre-eclampsia.

Extensive thermal injury to the red cells of patients with severe burns may produce a picture of fragmentation haemolysis with many small spherocytes and crenated cells.

'Toxic' Haemolysis

The exotoxin of *Clostridium welchii* may produce a life-threatening haemolysis with characteristic tiny spherocytes in the blood film. A similar picture may be seen in response to certain snake venoms. The pathogenesis of haemolytic anaemia in malaria is complex, including parasite-induced cell lysis, immune haemolysis, stimulation of the reticulo-endothelial system, dyserythropoiesis and hypersplenism. Falciparum malaria may be accompanied by disseminated intravascular coagulation and severe intravascular haemolysis ('blackwater fever').

Chemicals capable of causing haemolysis include copper and arsenic.

Haemolysis Due to Other Changes in the Red Cell Environment

In chronic liver disease, the abnormal lipid composition of the blood results in excessive incorporation of cholesterol in the red cell membrane. The mildest change is target cell formation due to an increased surface area to volume ratio, but in severe liver disease the red cells become rigid and are destroyed in passage through the microcirculation (especially in the spleen). Severe haemolysis in liver disease is a poor prognostic sign (*see* Chapter 25).

A degree of haemolysis is common in patients with chronic renal failure and may occasionally be exacerbated by haemodialysis. The precise toxin which accumulates in renal failure is uncertain.

FURTHER READING

Rosse W. F. (1981). The acquired haemolytic anaemias. In *Postgraduate Haematology* (Hoffbrand A. V., Lewis S. M., eds.). London: Heinemann Medical Books, pp. 229–268.

Chapter Six

The Haemoglobinopathies

DEFINITION

The term haemoglobinopathy describes inherited abnormalities of one or more of the four globin chains in haemoglobin. The thalassaemias are those disorders where the rate of synthesis is slow, but the structure of the chains produced is normal. In the structural variants, such as sickle-cell diseases, the amino acid sequence of globin is abnormal, frequently with only a single substitution. A third type of disorder, hereditary persistence of fetal haemoglobin, results from failure of the switch from fetal to adult haemoglobin production which normally occurs shortly after birth (*see* Table 6.1).

BACKGROUND

Normal adult haemoglobin is made of four haem molecules nestling in two pairs of α- and β-chains of globin. In the fetus and

Table 6.1
CLASSIFICATION OF HAEMOGLOBINOPATHIES

Abnormality	Examples
Reduced rate of chain synthesis	Thalassaemias, e.g. α- and β-thalassaemias
Abnormal chains (amino acid alterations)	Structural variants, e.g. HbS, HbC
Failure of switch from HbF to HbA	Hereditary persistence of fetal haemoglobin (HPFH)

Hb = haemoglobin.

newborn, a pair of γ-chains combines with the α-chains. Structural abnormalities in the amino acid composition and sequence may give rise to instability or to abnormal oxygen transport (*see* Table 6.2). The instability may result in a haemolytic anaemia, sometimes drug-induced, or to tissue damage caused by blocking of small vessels by abnormally stiff red cells. The rare abnormalities in oxygen transport may lead to congenital cyanosis if the oxygen affinity is low or if the haem pocket is abnormal (resulting in production of methaemoglobinaemia) or to polycythaemia if the oxygen affinity is abnormally high.

Inheritance

The inheritance is autosomal and co-dominant. Where one of a pair of globin chains is abnormal, the person is usually clinically well and is said to be heterozygous or to have the 'trait' (e.g. sickle-cell trait). Where both chains are abnormal, the patient is homozygous and is said to have the disease (e.g. sickle-cell disease). Distinction between these states is extremely important, but often not recognized by the family. Mixed disorders with different abnormalities, sometimes affecting different globin chains, lead to a great variety of conditions, and family studies may be needed for diagnosis.

Table 6.2
TYPES OF CLINICAL PROBLEMS CAUSED BY STRUCTURAL HAEMOGLOBIN VARIANTS

Clinical problem	*Examples*
Infarction	Sickle-cell disease and HbSC disease
Chronic haemolysis	HbC disease and unstable haemoglobins
Drug-induced haemolysis	Some unstable haemoglobins, e.g. Hb Zurich
Thalassaemia-like	HbE and Hb Constant Spring
Congenital cyanosis	Low affinity haemoglobins and HbMs
Congenital polycythaemia	High affinity haemoglobins

Hb = haemoglobin.

Incidence

The inherited disorders of globin are the commonest single gene disorders in the world, with hundreds of millions of thalassaemic or sickle cell heterozygotes. The advantage in survival resulting from resistance to malaria is probably the main reason for the persistence of the abnormalities, and the price for this advantage is the yearly birth of one quarter of a million severely affected homozygotes.

Geography

The geography of each disorder is described later, but it should be emphasized that, with modern travel and migrations, physicians everywhere must be competent to deal with the exacting needs of patients suffering from the more serious disorders.

THE THALASSAEMIAS

Definition

The thalassaemias are autosomal co-dominant hereditary disorders with impaired synthetic rates of one or more of the globin chains of haemoglobin. The chains are structurally normal, but the defect leads to ineffective erythropoiesis, haemolysis, microcytosis and anaemia.

Incidence and Geography

Thalassaemia is extremely common, with about 100 million people affected, of whom over 80 per cent are in Asia. About 40 000 children with thalassaemia major are born yearly, while some 20 000 babies are stillborn or die shortly after birth from α-thalassaemia. The term thalassaemia derives from the Greek word for sea and reflects the fact that the disorder was originally recognized in a broad belt around the Mediterranean, but both α and β disorders are found extending from here through the Middle East and the Indian subcontinent to South East Asia, and as far south in Africa as Nigeria (Figs. 6.1 and 6.2—all figures are

56 *Clinical Haematology*

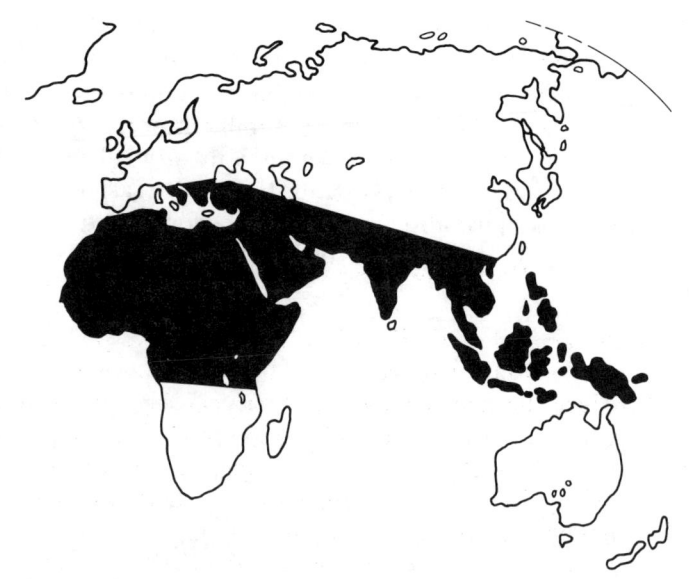

Fig. 6.1. Alpha-thalassaemia. Old World distribution. (Maps modified from Fleming 1987, with permission).

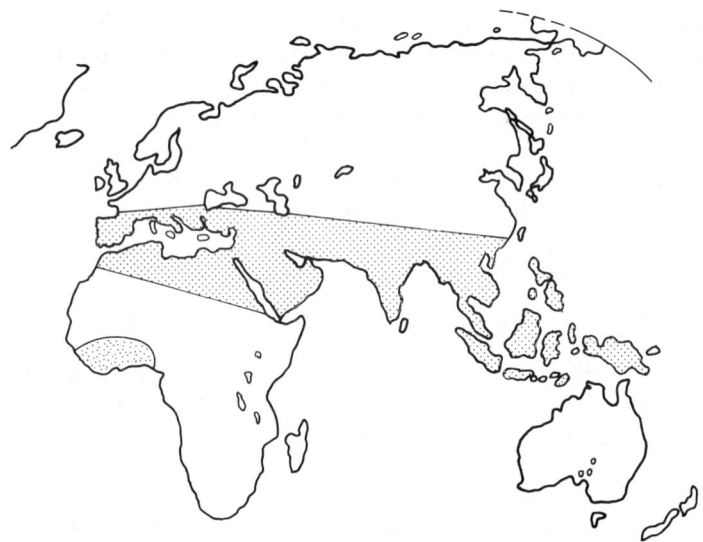

Fig. 6.2. Beta-thalassaemia. Old World distribution.

modified from Fleming 1987, with permission). Up to 30 per cent of the population in parts of the Mediterranean are found to have β-thalassaemia trait. In the UK, the indigenous population is not exempt from the trait, and with greater migration, the disorders may present to the physician anywhere in the world.

Pathology and Genetics

Normal adult haemoglobin (HbA) has two α- and two β-chains of globin. In the thalassaemias, reduction of synthesis of one type of chain will reduce the haemoglobin synthesis, causing microcytosis and resulting in an excess of the other type of chain. These free chains are unstable and precipitate, causing shortened red cell precursor survival (ineffective erythropoiesis) or shortened red cell survival (haemolytic anaemia). The marrow attempts to compensate for the anaemia, giving rise in the more severe disorders to marked expansion of the marrow cavity (producing bone abnormalities) and to extramedullary erythropoiesis in the liver and spleen.

Alpha-thalassaemia

Synthesis of α-chains is controlled by four genes, two from each parent on chromosome 16, and the severity of thalassaemia increases in proportion to the number of these genes which are affected. A variant commonly associated with α-thalassaemia is a structural abnormality of the α-chain, where there is a mutation of the normal terminating codon so that the chain is elongated by 31 amino acids. This variant, known as haemoglobin Constant Spring, behaves clinically like a gene deletion, with impaired synthetic rates of the α-chain.

Beta-thalassaemia

Synthesis of β-chains is controlled by two genes, one from each parent on chromosome 11. Defects may result in impaired (β^+-thalassaemia) or absent (β^0-thalassaemia) chain synthesis. Again, the clinical severity reflects the degree of impairment, which is genetically controlled. A structural abnormality of the β-chains, giving rise to haemoglobin Lepore (a hybrid of parts of the β- and δ-chains), clinically resembles the other β-thalassaemias (*see* Table 6.3).

Table 6.3
CLINICAL AND ELECTROPHORETIC FINDINGS IN THE β-THALASSAEMIAS

Chains	Homozygote	Heterozygote
β	Thalassaemia major Severe microcytic anaemia and haemolysis Only HbF and HbA$_2$ present, but some HbA in less severe variety (β$^+$)	Thalassaemia minor Mild microcytic anaemia HbA$_2$ > 3·5%
δβ	Thalassaemia intermedia Moderate haemolytic anaemia HbF only	Thalassaemia minor HbF 5–15%, HbA$_2$ normal
δβ fusion (Hb Lepore)	Thalassaemia major or Thalassaemia intermedia HbF and Hb Lepore	Thalassaemia minor Hb Lepore 5–15%, HbA$_2$ normal

INTERACTION BETWEEN THALASSAEMIAS AND STRUCTURAL HAEMOGLOBINOPATHIES

Disorder	Findings
Sickle β-thalassaemia	
HbS + β$^+$-thalassaemia	Mild disease (common in Negroes)
HbS + β^0-thalassaemia	Severe, as sickle-cell disease (common in Mediterranean regions)
HbC thalassaemia	
HbC + β$^+$-thalassaemia	Mild haemolysis and splenomegaly Target cells on blood film (West Africa)
HbE thalassaemia	
HbE + β^0-thalassaemia	Severe, as thalassaemia major (South-East Asia and India)

Hb = haemoglobin.

Molecular Basis

In most α-thalassaemias, the gene coding for the chain is absent. The β-thalassaemias are extremely heterogeneous, and may involve gene deletions, nonsense mutations (leading to termination of reading too early or too late), frameshifts, abnormalities at the intron/extron junction (leading to splicing abnormalities), abnormalities further upstream from the gene (leading to problems of regulation), or abnormalities of transcription.

The genetics have been extensively studied in thalassaemia and have proved excellent models for understanding human gene regulation. A particular advantage has been the ready availability of messenger RNA from reticulocytes in blood. Using reverse transcriptase, this can be copied to DNA and followed by hybridization, cloning, cutting (using restriction endonucleases), joining (using DNA ligases) and other analytical techniques.

Clinical Presentation and Investigation

Alpha-thalassaemias

Both fetal haemoglobin (haemoglobin F) and adult haemoglobin (haemoglobin A) contain two α-globin chains, combined in the former case with two γ-chains and in the latter with two β-chains. Abnormalities in α-chains may be expected to affect all ages. Tetramers of γ-chains (haemoglobin Barts) in the newborn, or tetramers of β-chains (haemoglobin H) later on, may be found.

In the most severe form (hydrops foetalis), where all four genes are affected, no haemoglobin F can be produced and most of the haemoglobin is haemoglobin Barts. The baby is stillborn prematurely or dies shortly after birth. Pre-eclampsia and toxaemia are common.

Where three genes are affected (haemoglobin H disease), a moderate microcytic anaemia is usual, with haemoglobin levels of 7 to 10 g/dl; patients are prone to infections. At birth, haemoglobin Barts is easily shown, and after about six months of age, when the normal switch from fetal to adult haemoglobin should occur, haemoglobin H levels of about 10 per cent are found, and plentiful precipitates from free β-chains can be shown as inclusions in the red cells by staining with vital stains such as cresyl blue.

Where two genes are affected (α-thalassaemia trait), there is usually no clinical problem, but the blood may show a mild microcytic anaemia. Confirmation is often difficult and may require repeat and prolonged examinations for the occasional red cells showing precipitated globin by vital stains. Chain synthesis rates or DNA analysis may be needed for diagnosis.

Where only one gene is involved (silent α-thalassaemia), the diagnosis is least difficult at birth, when about one per cent levels of haemoglobin Barts can be found.

Beta-thalassaemias

β-chains are not found in fetal haemoglobin, and so no blood disorder is seen until the baby is over six months old, when the switch to adult haemoglobin takes effect.

In β-thalassaemia trait, there is usually a mild and asymptomatic microcytic anaemia with haemoglobin levels above 9 g/dl, but these levels may fall, particularly in pregnancy. Diagnosis is suspected from the marked microcytosis in relation to the haemoglobin level, e.g. haemoglobin 10 g/dl and mean corpuscular haemoglobin (MCH) 20 pg or mean corpuscular volume (MCV) 60 fl, from the minimal anisocytosis and from the plentiful target cells. It is confirmed by finding a haemoglobin A_2 level greater than 3·5 per cent. If there is concurrent iron deficiency, haemoglobin A_2 levels will be lower than expected. Haemoglobin F levels are of no great help except for genetic studies—they may be normal or slightly increased.

Beta-thalassaemia major is inherited in simple Mendelian fashion, statistically affecting one in four children of parents who both have the trait. It is a severe disorder, with progressive anaemia developing after six months of age, and usually leads to death at under three years if untreated. Ninety per cent of developing erythroblasts are destroyed before becoming red cells (ineffective erythropoiesis), and those that escape the marrow are bizarre and have a short survival. The child shows the classic triad of haemolysis with anaemia, jaundice and splenomegaly, and suffers from heart failure, respiratory problems and failure to thrive. Infection may lead to drastic falls in the haemoglobin level. Expansion of the marrow by gross erythroid hyperplasia gives rise to a typical mongoloid facies with prominent cheek bones and to dental problems with malocclusion. Radiology shows a 'hair-on-end' appearance of the skull and expansion of the marrow cavity of long bones, sometimes subject to repeated fractures. The blood film may show many nucleated red cells, although reticulocyte counts may not be particularly raised. Extreme poikilocytosis and hypochromia are usual, and electrophoresis of haemoglobin shows reduced or absent haemoglobin A, with greatly increased haemoglobin F to compensate. Diagnosis at birth may be difficult, but is easy at three months of age.

Thalassaemia major, minor and intermedia

These are clinical terms denoting the severity of thalassaemia. Thalassaemia major is a severe transfusion-dependent anaemia, such as homozygous β-thalassaemia. Thalassaemia minor refers to the symptomless carrier states of α- or β-thalassaemias. Thalassaemia intermedia is a more confusing term applied to thalassaemias of various genetic forms (e.g. homozygous δβ-thalassaemia), where the clinical presentation is of intermediate severity, often presenting well after infancy with a haemolytic anaemia and splenomegaly. Long-term survival is usual, and problems with gallstones and leg ulcers have time to develop. Haemochromatosis is a common complication secondary to increased iron absorption, and is exacerbated if iron deficiency is diagnosed erroneously or if repeated transfusions are needed.

Family Studies

In many situations in thalassaemia, careful family studies are needed to elucidate the diagnosis fully, and this can be very difficult where there are mixtures of different chain abnormalities (which can partly balance each other), or combinations of thalassaemias with structural haemoglobinopathies.

Treatment

The milder forms of thalassaemia require no treatment, but accurate diagnosis is important if unnecessary iron therapy is to be avoided and if genetic counselling and antenatal diagnosis is contemplated.

With intermediate cases, transfusion should be given only if there is severe anaemia with growth failure, and measures to avoid iron overload should be considered. Folate needs are increased and supplements usually given. Infections should be treated promptly, and anaemia monitored in pregnancy.

Thalassaemia major is a challenging problem for good management, both of the child and of the family. High-transfusion regimens, using filtered or processed red cells, are now fashionable, aiming to keep the haemoglobin levels above 9 g/dl in order to minimize marrow output of the abnormal cells. Splenectomy may be needed if hypersplenism increases transfusion requirements, but it is delayed if possible until the child is over five years old. The quality of life of such children is greatly improved compared with the earlier minimal transfusion regimens, which were designed to restrict iron overload but resulted in recurrent heart failure, infections, repeated admissions, failure to thrive and early death. With high-transfusion regimens, the problem of iron overload leads to death from heart failure and cirrhosis in the late teens, but iron chelation therapy could improve this. At present the chelation is extremely expensive and involves daily subcutaneous infusions of desferrioxamine, usually given as an overnight infusion using a pump. Complications include yersinia infection, unexpected fatalities and the development of cataracts, which should be monitored by annual ophthalmic checks. Cheaper and effective oral agents will, it is hoped, soon be available. In Italy, where experience is greatest, bone marrow transplantation in infancy is having some success as a radical treatment.

Prevention

If heterozygotes avoided marrying other heterozygotes, their children could not inherit the severe homozygous diseases. Pilot trials along these lines are not looking successful to date because counselling does not modify behaviour.

Antenatal diagnosis

In high technology countries, antenatal screening programs are common. Blood of patients at risk is tested for thalassaemia trait at diagnosis of their first pregnancy, and if positive, the child's father is tested without delay. If he has the same disorder, the problem is discussed with the family with a view to testing the fetus for the homozygous condition (a one-in-four chance) and to early abortion if the condition is found. A diagnosis is now possible from about nine weeks of pregnancy by chorionic villous sampling and DNA analysis. It should, of course, be stressed that in three out of four such tests, the baby is found not to be severely affected and the pregnancy continues with no anxieties.

THE SICKLING DISORDERS

The sickling disorders account for the vast majority of the clinically important structural disorders, and the great majority of them are found in Negroes from Africa, with small numbers in the Mediterranean, Middle East and India. Sickle-cell haemoglobin, haemoglobin S, differs from normal adult haemoglobin A in that the normal sixth amino acid, glutamic acid, is replaced by valine.

Varieties

Sickle-cell trait is the heterozygous state for haemoglobin S, where the haemoglobin consists of a mixture of haemoglobins A and S. The homozygous state is called sickle-cell disease and consists of haemoglobin S with no haemoglobin A. Mixed heterozygous disorders with haemoglobins S and C (haemoglobin SC disease) and with haemoglobin S and β-thalassaemia are also common and important, but many other combinations have been described.

Sickle-Cell Trait

About 60 million people, mostly African Negroes, have the trait. There are no clinical features, and the blood film and haemoglobin levels are normal. However, under conditions of severe oxygen deprivation (Po_2 under 2·66 kPa, or 20 mmHg), as in unpressurized high altitude flight, poor anaesthesia or severe pneumonia, the infarctive crises typical of sickle-cell anaemia may develop. Recurrent haematuria may occur, and the kidney may show a poor ability to concentrate urine. It has been reported that Negro soldiers with the trait are more likely to suffer sudden death than others under severe field exercises.

Patients from these areas should have their blood screened before surgery by haemoglobin electrophoresis. In the sickling test, a drop of blood on a glass slide is mixed with a reducing agent such as sodium metabisulphate, sealed and examined for sickle cells an hour later. A simple test is the sickle solubility test, which can be performed in about five minutes (but is not considered to be entirely reliable). In both these tests, negative results imply the absence of a sickling disorder, whereas positive results are found in all sickling disorders, whatever their severity. A positive result with a normal haemoglobin level is very suggestive of the trait, but haemoglobin electrophoresis is needed for confirmation. This shows over 50 per cent haemoglobin A and smaller amounts of haemoglobin S, which runs more slowly because of the valine substitution.

Adequate oxygenation and hydration is important with surgery, but it is also important not to label these patients as abnormal, as they have a completely normal span and quality of life.

Sickle-Cell Disease

Sickle-cell disease is found in one to two per cent of births in parts of Africa, and about 100 000 people are born yearly with this disorder worldwide (Fig. 6.3). In 1988, some 4000 people in the UK have sickle-cell disease, and more than 70 babies are born with the disease annually.

Clinical presentation

The clinical severity of sickle-cell disease varies considerably from one family to another, and particularly mild forms are found where haemoglobin F levels are high. The severity also changes greatly from one country to another; death in childhood is common in under-developed countries with poor nutrition and tropical infections, whereas survival to old age is more usual in developed countries.

While anaemia is usually marked (haemoglobin around 7 g/dl, although occasionally normal levels may be found), it causes far fewer clinical problems than might be expected because the oxygen affinity is low, resulting in good release of oxygen to the tissues. Children under 10 years of age usually show the signs of a haemolytic anaemia, with anaemia, variable jaundice and spleno-

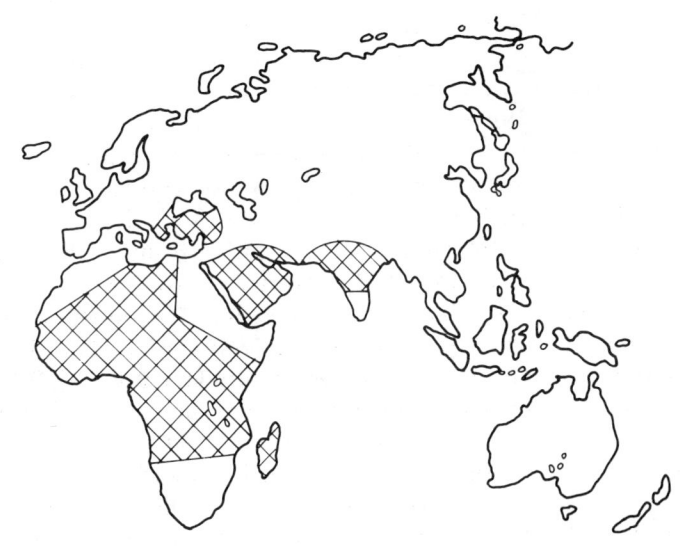

Fig. 6.3. Haemoglobin S. Old World distribution.

megaly. In older children, the spleen is usually impalpable because, over a period of time, repeated infarctive episodes result in a shrunken fibrotic spleen. Indeed, a palpable spleen at this stage should suggest consideration of alternative diagnoses, such as sickle thalassaemia or haemoglobin SC disease. The splenic loss leads to the usual features of hyposplenism in the blood film (*see* Chapter 12) and to increased risks of pyogenic infection, particularly pneumococcal and meningococcal infections.

The hallmark of sickle-cell disease is one of recurrent crises (*see* Table 6.4). The commonest are 'infarctive (or painful) crises' caused by the rigidity of red cells in the reduced state blocking small vessels. This can happen with the oxygen pressures normally found in the tissues (Po_2 5·32 kPa, or 40 mmHg). Once the blood is slowed, the process enters a vicious circle, with stasis leading to deoxygenation and further rigidity and stasis. Once started, the process therefore becomes extremely hard to reverse. The crisis may be precipitated by infection or dehydration and may last for any length of time between two days and over a week, often requiring strong analgesics. In some patients, crises may occur every two weeks or so, whereas others may have crises every few years. They tend to become less frequent with age. In children under three years old, the bones of the hands and feet are prone to

Table 6.4
SICKLE CELL CRISES

Crisis	Salient features
Infarctive	Often painful (bone, abdomen, joint, CNS, lung), Hb stable
	In girdle syndrome, lung, liver and mesentery all involved
Haemolytic	Hb falls, reticulocyte count high (may complicate above)
Sequestration	Hb falls, reticulocyte count high, liver and spleen enlarge
Aplastic	Hb falls, reticulocyte count low (commonly parvovirus)

CNS = central nervous system; Hb = haemoglobin.

infarction causing painful dactylis (hand–foot syndrome), and epiphyseal damage may lead to shortening of individual digits. Later in life, the sites may include the abdomen (presenting as an acute abdomen, sometimes with quiet bowel sounds and invariably with the raised white cell count and pyrexia found in infarctive crises), joints and muscles, penis (priapism), chest (presenting with pleuritic pain, but sometimes rapidly developing into the acute chest syndrome with life-threatening anoxia and anaemia from pulmonary vessel blockage), and nervous system (fits, hemiplegia, coma, optic nerve problems and local signs). Diagnosis of painful crises is usually easy but can be very difficult, as the pains may start insidiously and may have a bizarre distribution in the back, bones or muscles, suggesting a psychogenic origin.

Three other types of crisis are found. The 'sequestration crisis' occurs mostly in young children and is potentially lethal. The child presents with rapid onset of progressive anaemia, and the spleen and liver enlarge rapidly and painfully as most of the circulating blood is trapped in them. Repeated attacks are common. A particularly severe form of crisis is called the girdle syndrome and involves infarction in the lungs, liver and mesentery, with severe back pain, anoxia, growing liver and silent bowel. 'Aplastic crises', often secondary to parvovirus infection, result in a rapid fall in haemoglobin levels without other clinical findings. The reticulocyte count is low, which distinguishes this condition from those described above and also from the rather rare 'haemolytic crisis' with marked haemolysis complicating a painful crisis.

More chronic problems include progressive infarctive damage to tissues with poor collateral circulation. The humeral and femoral heads may become necrotic over a period of time, with gross deformities. Surprisingly, the infarctive episodes can be completely silent, and routine radiology has shown severe joint damage in patients with no history of hip pain. The eye is vulnerable to a proliferative retinitis, with blindness an end result. The heart usually shows a functional (anaemic) murmur, and acute strain is seen with the lung syndrome. In Africa and the West Indies, chronic leg ulceration is common, and older patients may develop pigment gallstones.

Pregnancy may be complicated by more frequent crises, and management should be jointly by obstetrician and haematologist. The baby is at considerable risk of prematurity and increased mortality.

Investigation

The blood usually shows marked anaemia (haemoglobin 7 g/dl), but this is functionally mild because the oxygen affinity is reduced (P_{50} of 40–60 mmHg, compared with a normal P_{50} of 30 mmHg). Reticulocytes are increased (10–15 per cent) and target cells prominent. Sickle cells may be hard to find in patients with few irreversibly sickled cells, but usually they are frequent, correlating with the shortening of red cell survival. Signs of hyposplenism are seen in older children and adults. The sickling test, needed when sickles are not seen on the plain blood film, is positive and electrophoresis shows no haemoglobin A at all, but mainly haemoglobin S with some haemoglobin F (5 per cent or more). Care with interpretation of results is needed in transfused patients.

At birth, only small amounts of haemoglobin A are found in patients with sickle-cell trait. Its detection by a sensitive method (e.g. electrophoresis on acid citrate agar) excludes a diagnosis of sickle-cell disease. It is important to test for maternal blood contamination if cord blood is being examined, and if any abnormality is found, it is wise to confirm the diagnosis at about three months of age.

Prognosis

In the West, there is still a high death rate in the first year of life and this emphasizes the importance of early diagnosis. With better care in the early years, children may escape the high early mortality from pneumococcal infections and sequestration crises and grow to suffer painful infarctive crises, with a near normal survival.

Treatment

Good nutrition and general health clearly affect the course of the disease. Folic acid supplementation is wise, as the needs are increased because of the chronic haemolysis. Rapid treatment of infections is important in reducing the likelihood of painful crises, and many authors advocate prophylactic treatment with oral penicillin as soon as the diagnosis is made (ideally at about six weeks old), to reduce the high early mortality. Where possible, the patient should be managed by a team with special interest in the disorder.

The painful crisis usually requires admission for copious hydration (particularly important as the kidneys are impaired and cannot concentrate urine), treatment of any suspected infection, and immediate and adequate analgesics (often with frequent pethidine). Adequate explanation of the problem and the patient's confidence in the medical team are important in the management of a patient in severe pain. Oxygen is needed in the respiratory crisis, but is of doubtful value in other cases. Transfusion is seldom needed, but in the sequestration crisis, urgent transfusion and frequent monitoring of the haemoglobin concentration is essential to keep up with the decline. Exchange transfusion may be life-saving with the lung or girdle syndrome and neurological crises, and should be considered for serious crises which do not settle with conservative treatment (e.g. haemoglobin falling below 5 g/dl, arterial Po_2 below 8 kPa or absent bowel sounds for three days). Elective exchange transfusions are used before major surgery (during which tourniquets and anoxia must be avoided, maintaining the arterial Po_2 above 16 kPa, or 120 mmHg), and have been successful for recurrent severe crises and for priapism not settling within 24 hours. Their place in pregnancy complicated by frequent crises or severe anaemia is still debatable, disappointing results being attributed to the achievement of inadequate (under 70 per cent) haemoglobin A levels. Regular transfusion regimens will carry the risks of transmission of infection and production of antibodies, and so these risks must be balanced against any potential advantages (*see* Chapters 14 and 28).

Community surveys with a view to genetic counselling can result in the unnecessary labelling of people as 'sicklers', resulting in inappropriate difficulties with jobs and insurance. However, in the UK, the Department of Health and Social Security (DHSS) is now recommending that people who have been tested for haemoglobinopathies should be encouraged to carry cards showing the results. Antenatal diagnosis should be considered only where the disorder running in the family is severe.

Sickle C Disease

This disease is found in Negro populations coming from West Africa, particularly west of the River Niger (*see* Table 6.4). The molecular abnormality of haemoglobin C is a substitution of the sixth amino acid, glutamic acid, by lysine.

Clinical presentation

The clinical problems are similar to those of sickle-cell disease, but with fewer painful crises and more thrombotic problems. The haemolytic anaemia is mild, but the spleen usually remains large after childhood—a point of difference from sickle-cell disease. Clinical problems often do not appear until adulthood and largely relate to infrequent infarctive problems. Avascular necrosis of the femoral or humeral head is common and results from repeated small infarcts, which may be asymptomatic until considerable bone damage has occurred, when pain and limitation of movement become a progressive and difficult problem. Blindness may develop after retinitis proliferans or retinal detachment. Pregnancy is usually uneventful, but some patients show increased infarctive problems, particularly in the lungs near and shortly after delivery. The high haemoglobin compared with sickle-cell disease may contribute to these problems.

Investigation

The haemoglobin is usually only slightly reduced (10–12 g/dl), reflecting the minimal reduction in oxygen affinity (P_{50} of 40 mmHg), and the reticulocyte count only slightly raised. The MCV tends to be low and the mean corpuscular haemoglobin concentration (MCHC) high, which reflects the blood film appearance with many targets, frequent small dense cells (with crystals) and only occasional sickles. The sickling and solubility tests are positive. Electrophoresis shows no haemoglobin A, but both haemoglobins S and C. Haemoglobin S runs slowly because of the loss of negative charge of glutamic acid by neutral valine, and haemoglobin C runs even slower because of the positive charge of its lysine substitution.

Treatment

This should follow similar lines to the treatment for sickle-cell disease. In pregnancy, it is usual to anticoagulate near term to reduce the risk of thrombotic problems. If past pregnancies have been difficult or if major infarctive problems develop, exchange transfusions every four weeks or so from the twentieth week onwards, aimed at achieving haemoglobin A levels of over 60 to 70 per cent, have been advocated, but with conflicting evidence of success. The potential harmful effects of transfusion, particularly in Africa where human immunodeficiency virus (HIV) is a huge problem, have not been adequately stressed.

Sickle β-thalassaemia

This disease is uncommon (4000 sufferers worldwide), being found in North Africa, the Mediterranean, the Middle East and India, the Caribbean and the Americas. The findings are predictable. Where the thalassaemia defect is severe, with very reduced or absent globin chain production, the picture is hard to distinguish (without family studies) from sickle-cell disease. Where the defect is less severe, a mild version of sickle-cell disease is found, with moderate anaemia and haemolysis, splenomegaly, hypochromia and target and sickle cells on the blood film, and the presence of haemoglobin A in addition to haemoglobins S and F on electrophoresis. Unlike sickle-cell trait, the haemoglobin S is greater than 50 per cent.

Homozygous Haemoglobin C Disease

This is a mild disorder, requiring no treatment. There is slight anaemia and splenomegaly, the blood film is dominated by target cells, and electrophoresis shows the very slow moving haemoglobin C with a little haemoglobin F.

THE UNSTABLE HAEMOGLOBINS

In these very rare hereditary disorders, a structural change in a globin chain renders haemoglobin liable to precipitate in the red cells or precursors. A mild haemolytic anaemia with splenomegaly and a predisposition to pigment gallstones are usual. Acute haemolysis may be induced by oxidative drugs, such as sulphonamides.

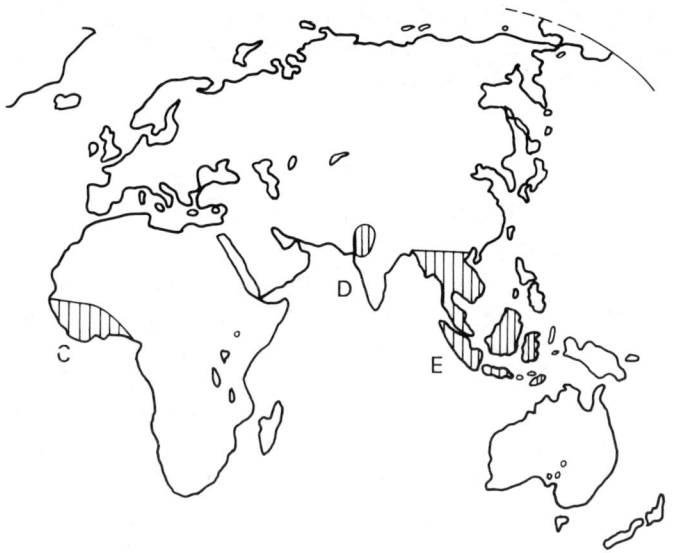

Fig. 6.4. Haemoglobins C, D and E. Old World distribution.

THE HAEMOGLOBIN Ms

In these extremely rare disorders, substitutions around the haem pocket result in oxidation of haemoglobin to methaemoglobin. This is extremely poor in transporting oxygen and results in cyanosis—from birth in the α-chain disorders and a little later in the β-chain disorders. With levels of methaemoglobin above 20 per cent, symptoms of oxygen shortage (such as those of severe anaemia) may be found. The family history is usually positive, and diagnosis (once the disease is considered) is simple. The Po_2 is normal and spectroscopy shows increased methaemoglobin with an abnormal peak. Haemoglobin electrophoresis under specific conditions is abnormal.

In patients with central cyanosis, the differential diagnosis is between anoxia and the rare methaemoglobinaemias or the even rarer low affinity haemoglobins (*see* below). In anoxia, the arterial Po_2 is low and the blood blue as in venous blood. In the methaemoglobins, the Po_2 is normal, and the blood appears brown when taken into a syringe. The presence of even small amounts of methaemoglobin can be shown by spectroscopic methods. The differential diagnosis of methaemoglobinaemia includes oxidative drug overdosage (e.g. phenacetin, potassium perchlorate—weed killer) and NADH reductase deficiency (where there is cyanosis from birth, a normal methaemoglobin peak and reduced enzyme assays).

Treatment with ascorbic acid or methylene blue is of no help. Most patients remain well if oxidative drugs are avoided.

THE HIGH AFFINITY HAEMOGLOBINOPATHIES

In these rare disorders, the affinity of haemoglobin for oxygen is abnormally high. They should be suspected whenever polycythaemia develops from childhood. Diagnosis may be difficult because haemoglobin electrophoresis is often normal, and oxygen dissociation studies are needed to measure the affinity. If the P_{50} is reduced, detailed haemoglobin analysis should confirm the diagnosis. No treatment is needed, but if there are thrombotic problems from vascular disease, venesection may be appropriate.

THE LOW AFFINITY HAEMOGLOBINS

This rare type of disorder leads to central cyanosis with normal oxygen tensions and with adequate oxygenation of tissues, despite the anaemia and cyanosis.

FURTHER READING

Fleming A. F. (1987). Anaemia as a world health problem. In *Oxford Textbook of Medicine*, 2nd edn. Oxford: Oxford University Press, pp. 19.72–19.75.

Serjeant G. R. (1985). *Sickle Cell Disease*. Oxford: Oxford University Press.

Weatherall D.J., Clegg J.B. (1981). *The Thalassaemia Syndromes*, 3rd edn. Oxford: Blackwell Scientific Publications.

Chapter Seven

Neutropenia

Neutropenia is diagnosed by finding a total neutrophil count of less than $1.5 \times 10^9/l$. This chapter will discuss only 'isolated' neutropenia, i.e. in the absence of anaemia or thrombocytopenia. Isolated neutropenia is relatively uncommon. It may be present in Blacks and Yemenite Jews, or it may be secondary to drugs, infections, auto-immune or iso-immune phenomena, or cyclic fluctuations of white cell production (cyclic neutropenia).

BLACKS AND YEMENITE JEWS

Persistent neutropenia is frequently present in African and West Indian Blacks. A similar syndrome is present in Yemenite Jewish people. The pathophysiology is unclear, but current information would favour either a defective release of neutrophils from the marrow or increased margination of these cells in the vascular channels. The neutropenia may be quite severe but rarely gives rise to clinical problems, and in fact, infection may be accompanied by a rising neutrophil count.

DRUG-INDUCED NEUTROPENIA

Many, if not all, drugs are potentially capable of producing neutropenia (*see* Table 7.1).

The mechanisms of action fall into three broad categories:

1. Dose-related, e.g. chemotherapeutic agents
2. Immune-mediated, e.g. amidopyrine
3. Idiosyncratic, e.g. phenothiazines.

Table 7.1
DRUGS CAUSING NEUTROPENIA*

Phenothiazines
Sulphonamides
Chloramphenicol
Phenylbutazone
Amidopyrine
Carbimazole
Chemotherapeutic agents

*These are examples, and not a complete list of drugs associated with neutropenia.

INFECTIONS

Severe neutropenia may occur in Gram-negative septicaemia with endotoxaemia. Bacterial and protozoal infections, such as typhoid, paratyphoid, brucellosis and malaria, may be associated with reduced circulating neutrophil counts. Neutropenia may be found in patients with viral infections, such as infectious mononucleosis, influenza, rubella and acute hepatitis.

IMMUNE-MEDIATED NEUTROPENIA

Iso-immune neutropenia may occur in neonates following the transplacental passage of neutrophil-specific IgG antibodies from the mother. As with other neonatal iso-immune syndromes, improvement in neutrophil counts will parallel the natural decline in maternal IgG levels, usually from six to twelve weeks after birth.

Idiopathic auto-immune neutropenia is a rare disease in which auto-antibodies with specific affinity for neutrophil antigens are found. Severe neutropenia with recurrent bacterial infections may occur. Neutrophil counts frequently rise during a course of corticosteroids. Whether splenectomy should be used to treat such patients has yet to be determined. Both steroids and splenectomy should be used with caution because of their potential for increasing the risk of infection.

Felty's syndrome, characterized by rheumatoid arthritis, neutropenia and splenomegaly, typically occurs in long-standing 'burnt out' rheumatoid arthritis. The neutropenia, which may be severe, is thought to be auto-immune in type, as increased levels of neutrophil-associated antibody can be detected. The beneficial response to steroids and splenectomy would also favour an immune mechanism for this syndrome.

Neutropenia occurs in up to 50 per cent of patients with systemic lupus erythematosus. It is rarely severe, and therefore specific treatment is usually not required. An immune mechanism, with high levels of neutrophil-associated antibody, has been suggested. In this situation, an IgG antibody may cross the placenta and produce transient noenatal neutropenia.

CYCLIC NEUTROPENIA

Cyclic fluctuation of haemopoiesis is probably a normal event. In some individuals, however, cyclic fluctuations occurring, usually, every 21 days are associated with neutropenia, which may be severe and accompanied by recurrent bacterial infections. Some patients, however, with quite severe neutropenia do not seem unduly susceptible to infections. In such patients, an accompanying monocytosis may help to protect them. Treatment is usually not necessary, but responses have been reported to lithium, corticosteroids and recombinant granulocyte colony stimulating factor (G-CSF).

CLINICAL APPROACH TO THE NEUTROPENIC PATIENT

The risk of infection is directly related to the severity of the neutropenia. There is probably no increased susceptibility to infection should the neutrophil count be greater than $1 \times 10^9/l$. In neutropenic patients, prophylactic antibiotics should not be used. Their effectiveness in preventing infection has not been proven and they may increase a patient's susceptibility to opportunistic infections. There is conflicting evidence as to the value of such procedures as patient isolation and laminar flow facilities, except perhaps in the most severely neutropenic patients, e.g. following bone marrow transplantation. Strict handwashing between patients and other measures to reduce cross infection have been demonstrated to be effective in reducing the incidence of infection.

In neutropenic patients, the most common indicator of infection is an isolated pyrexia without any obvious infective focus. Transient bacteraemia in this situation usually arises endogenously, frequently by the passage of organisms through the mucosa of the gastro-intestinal tract. When this occurs, the patient requires immediate hospitalization, and treatment with broad spectrum, intravenous antibiotics should be instituted without delay. Investigations include blood cultures, urine culture, chest X-ray, examination of skin, mouth and throat, and inspection of the perineum and perianal regions. In most instances, the patient will respond to treatment within 72 hours. Prolonged fever, not responding to antibiotics, could be due to resistant bacterial or viral infections or, more worryingly, an opportunistic fungal infection.

As regards the cause of a patient's neutropenia, this may be obvious from the list outlined above. All drugs that the patient has been receiving should be discontinued where possible. Periodic white cell counts would confirm a diagnosis of cyclic neutropenia. Immune disorders may be identified by measuring neutrophil-associated immunoglobulin levels.

FURTHER READING

Williams W.J., Beutler E., Ersler A.J., Lichtman M.A., eds. (1986). *Haematology*. New York: McGraw-Hill.

Chapter Eight

Thrombocytopenia

DEFINITION

Thrombocytopenia is the reduction of the platelet count below $150 \times 10^9/l$ in a well collected sample of blood. When the count is below $80 \times 10^9/l$, abnormal bleeding may occur on trauma or surgery, and when the count is below $20 \times 10^9/l$, spontaneous haemorrhage is common.

AETIOLOGY

Reduction in the platelet count may reflect inadequate production from megakaryocytes in the marrow, or early destruction or removal in the circulation. In addition, massive red cell transfusion will result in a dilutional thrombocytopenia, because transfusions of stored blood contain no effective platelets (Table 8.1).

Marrow production of platelets will be reduced when the numbers of megakaryocytes are decreased by hypoplasia (sometimes drug-induced) or by replacement in leukaemias and other malignancies. Even with normal numbers of megakaryocytes, platelet production may be ineffective, and this is found with some drugs (e.g. thiazides), toxins (e.g. alcohol and virus infections), megaloblastic marrows and myelodysplasia.

Platelets may be removed prematurely from the circulation by destruction, consumption or sequestration by an enlarged spleen. Normal platelets survive for about 10 days in the circulation before removal by the reticulo-endothelial system. Premature destruction usually follows abnormal antibody coating of the platelets. Various types of antibodies are found. After viral infections, immune complexes may attach to the platelets causing transient thrombocytopenia. In chronic idiopathic thrombocyto-

Table 8.1
CAUSES OF THROMBOCYTOPENIA

Platelet production
  Megakaryocytes reduced
    Hypoplasia, e.g. drugs, radiation, congenital
    Infiltration by leukaemia, malignancy etc.
  Megakaryocytes dysplastic
    Drugs
    Toxins, e.g. alcohol
    Virus infections
    Megaloblastic marrow
    Myelodysplasia

Platelet removal
  Antibody-related
    Drug-induced antibodies
    Virus infection (immune complexes)
    ITP
    SLE and other collagen diseases
    Anti-Pl^{A1} (post-transfusion purpura and newborn)
  Hypersplenism
  Miscellaneous
    DIC
    HUS
    TTP
    Haemangioma

Platelet dilution
  High volume transfusion

DIC = disseminated intravascular coagulation; HUS = haemolytic uraemic syndrome; ITP = idiopathic thrombocytopenic purpura; SLE = systemic lupus erythematosus; TTP = thrombotic thrombocytopenia.

penic purpura (ITP), antibodies to platelets (which can sometimes be demonstrated in vitro) can cross the placenta, causing transient thrombocytopenia in the newborn. Similar antibodies to platelets may be found in auto-immune diseases, such as systemic lupus erythematosus (SLE). Antibodies to specific platelet antigens are responsible for the syndrome of post-transfusion purpura, in which patients who have previously been sensitized (usually multiparous women) develop sudden thrombocytopenia and bleeding 7–10 days after transfusion. The antibody involved is usually anti-Pl^{A1}, and the same antibody is involved in the rare cases of iso-immune neonatal thrombocytopenia, where the baby is Pl^{A1} antigen positive and the mother negative (analgous to Rhesus disease affecting the red cells). Another rare problem is that of drugs, such as quinine (e.g. in tonic water), inducing an antibody which acts against platelets only in the presence of the drug.

Consumption of platelets is often found in disseminated intravascular coagulation (DIC), where thrombi containing platelets and coagulation factors are formed in small vessels; the fall in platelet count is an indication of the severity of the problem. Platelet consumption may be mainly localized in the kidney in haemolytic uraemic syndrome (HUS), seen in children and in the puerperium, and in the brain in thrombotic thrombocytopenia (TTP). Very rarely, platelets may be consumed in large haemangiomas.

Splenic sequestration of platelets in hypersplenism usually causes mild thrombocytopenia (e.g. in liver disease), but on occasions, the thrombocytopenia can be severe. The spleen normally contains about 30 per cent of the body's platelets, but with splenic enlargement, it can increase to 90 per cent.

Incidence

Now that accurate platelet counts are performed routinely, it is realized that thrombocytopenia is extremely common, particularly drug- or virus-induced thrombocytopenia, and following major surgery with large volume transfusions.

SYMPTOMS AND SIGNS

Nature of the Bleeding Problem

The length of the bleeding history, including direct questions about bleeding problems following previous surgery, dental procedures or childbirth, should be established. Results of platelet counts on previous admissions can help, but counts in chronic ITP can fluctuate.

In mild thrombocytopenia, trauma or surgery are needed to provoke bleeding problems, but in severe thrombocytopenia, there is spontaneous bleeding and bruising. Platelets are needed for the primary arrest of haemorrhage and the clinical picture is distinct, with immediate and heavy bleeding from the skin and mucosal surfaces. The bleeding can often be stopped by pressure and does not tend to recur later. This contrasts with bleeding problems in the hereditary coagulation disorders, where spontaneous bleeding into joints and deep muscles and bleeding after dental extraction are characteristic, bleeding continuing intermittently for days.

Bleeding into the skin varies in severity from pin-point petechiae to larger purpura and to more extensive bruising (ecchymosis). Purpura is common in scratch marks and on the skin overlying the shins, and ecchymosis is often found at venepuncture sites. Mucosal bleeding commonly results in nose-bleeds, blood blisters in the mouth, gum bleeding, menorrhagia, and haematuria. Gastro-intestinal haemorrhage may lead to anaemia. Headaches, confusion or partial visual loss are worrying symptoms suggesting cerebral haemorrhage, but fundal haemorrhage may simply reflect severe anaemia, particularly in ITP.

General

A drug history should be taken with care, and exposure to chemicals considered. A history of a virus infection one or two weeks preceding the purpura is common in children with acute thrombocytopenia or with HUS, but in the latter, the child is often ill and will have renal impairment.

An iso-immune problem should be considered in a patient with a previously normal platelet count who develops thrombocytopenia about a week after transfusion. However, in this context, it is more common to find that drug therapy or even DIC is responsible.

Where thrombocytopenia is found in neonates, the mother should be reviewed for evidence of ITP or SLE (where the antibody may cross the placenta), or for evidence of 'TORCH' (intra-uterine infection from toxoplasma, rubella, cytomegalovirus or herpes). In seriously ill neonates, DIC with thrombocytopenia is not uncommon.

Examination for underlying disorders is always important, with the finding of splenomegaly against a diagnosis of ITP.

Acute Thrombocytopenic Purpura

Mild purpura of the skin and mouth with sudden onset about 10 days after a virus infection is common, particularly after mumps and rubella in children or infectious mononucleosis or respiratory infections in young adults. The course is usually short and treatment seldom needed. More than 90 per cent of cases show spontaneous remission within one year, but occasional deaths (much less than one per cent) have occurred from cerebral haemorrhage.

Chronic ITP

This is found more often in young adults, especially women. The onset is gradual, and there may be a past history of purpura. Patients may present with anaemia, rather than with a history of purpura or bleeding from other sites, and the nature of the problem may be recognized only when the blood count is checked. More typically, there is a history of bleeding, frequently from more than one site, and examination reveals scattered purpura. In general terms, about 10 per cent of patients have marked bleeding problems, and about 90 per cent have only minimal bleeding (even with platelet counts under $10 \times 10^9/l$). An enlarged spleen is unusual and suggests cirrhosis, lymphoma or some other underlying disorder. In Evans' syndrome, there is an associated auto-immune haemolytic anaemia.

INVESTIGATIONS

A good and reproducible bedside test of primary arrest of haemorrhage is the template bleeding time, provided that it is performed in a standardized manner. It is prolonged with thrombocytopenia and with disorders of platelet function, but is superfluous if there is obvious purpura. Hess's test (looking for purpura below an inflated sphygmomanometer cuff) is unreliable and seldom used now.

In marrow disorders with thrombocytopenia, the blood film often shows signs of an underlying disorder, e.g. pancytopenia in aplasia, abnormalities of the leucocytes in leukaemias, and macrocytosis with megaloblastic change. Isolated thrombocytopenia suggests ITP, drug-induced thrombocytopenia, or SLE. Anaemia and iron deficiency will occur if there is significant blood loss. Red cell fragmentation is common in patients with HUS, TTP or DIC, and in DIC a coagulation screen will be abnormal (*see* Chapter 13). Abnormal renal function is always present in HUS, and may be seen in TTP.

Marrow examination is essential and should include a trephine biopsy if a primary marrow disease is suspected. Typically, megakaryocyte numbers are low in hypoplastic disorders, normal but dysplastic in disorders of ineffective production, and increased and immature in disorders of increased destruction of platelets.

Unfortunately, tests for platelet antibodies in ITP and the immune thrombocytopenias are difficult, and reliable results are obtained in only a few specialist laboratories. In such laboratories, IgG, IgM or complement with activity to platelets can be shown in over 95 per cent of patients thought to have ITP. Positive results may also be found in patients with previous ITP whose platelet count has returned to normal, and occasionally in patients not thought to have immune problems. Given these limitations, it is generally acceptable to make the diagnosis of ITP without platelet antibody studies, but after exclusion of other causes (especially drugs and SLE).

In the thrombocytopenias caused by drug-induced antibodies against platelets, the antibody can be demonstrated in serum stored at presentation, but frequently the tests cannot be completed until the platelet count has recovered. Some patients have the lupus anticoagulant (Chapter 23).

DIFFERENTIAL DIAGNOSIS

The finding of an unexpectedly low platelet count in a patient with no obvious bleeding diathesis may suggest a poor venesection technique (where platelets are aggregated in small blood clots and therefore not counted) or a counting artefact due to platelet clumping (which can readily be seen in the blood film).

Telangiectasia and spider naevi blanch with pressure, whereas purpuric spots do not. Purpuric spots may be confused with early Campbell de Morgan's spots, but the latter tend to be raised and do not change with time, whereas purpuric spots start a bright pink colour and follow the familiar colour changes of bruises, turning purplish over the next few days and disappearing as the blood is reabsorbed, usually within a week.

Purpura and bleeding mucosal lesions in the presence of a normal platelet count suggest a platelet abnormality or, less commonly, a vascular abnormality, e.g. Henoch–Schönlein purpura.

SLE can present with thrombocytopenic purpura and is distinguished from ITP by measuring antinuclear factor (ANF) levels and DNA binding.

TREATMENT OF ITP

Intramuscular injections and aspirin-like drugs should be avoided, and it is helpful to put a reminder of this over the patient's bed.

While platelet therapy is usually contra-indicated in ITP (as the transfused platelets are destroyed by antibodies), it is important in the management of patients with marrow failure or DIC.

Treatment of acute thrombocytopenia in children is seldom necessary. Platelet transfusions are generally unhelpful, as the platelets are rapidly destroyed. Steroids are usually not needed but are often used in severe cases. Even platelet counts below $20 \times 10^9/l$ seldom cause life-threatening haemorrhage, and spontaneous recovery within a few weeks is usual.

Management of chronic ITP is controversial, but greater emphasis should always be placed on the degree of clinical bleeding rather than the platelet count. While some patients with counts below $10 \times 10^9/l$ have no bleeding problems (perhaps partly because the young large platelets released by the marrow are functionally very effective), others with counts over $20 \times 10^9/l$ can have serious bleeding problems. In general, there are no significant problems when the counts are over $50 \times 10^9/l$, and no treatment is needed.

Steroids are effective in the treatment of ITP. Their mode of action is complex and includes an effect on endothelial cells, phagocytic cells of the reticulo-endothelial system, antibody production and antigen–antibody binding. With counts below $50 \times 10^9/l$ and associated bleeding problems, it is usual to treat with prednisolone (about 60 mg daily). This may improve bleeding problems within a few days, even before the platelet count changes. The platelet count usually rises within one week, but delayed responses of up to four to six weeks occasionally occur. Even if patients respond rapidly, it is usual to maintain a high dose of steroids for about two weeks before gradual reduction. Although 80 per cent of patients will improve initially, the cure rate is only 20 per cent.

Splenectomy, which is usually avoided in young children, removes a major site of antibody production as well as the major site of platelet destruction. The mortality of the procedure (one to two per cent) is increased by prolonged steroid therapy, and so if the response to steroid therapy is unsatisfactory (i.e. the bleeding is not controlled or is controlled only on unacceptably high doses), splenectomy should not be delayed. The operation is often preceded by pneumococcal vaccination and followed by long-term oral penicillin. Bleeding problems at splenectomy are unusual, and the operation can, in general, be carried out without platelet cover. If bleeding does occur, platelet infusions should be delayed until after the splenic vessels are clamped. Some haematologists will attempt to boost the platelet count temporarily before surgery by a short course of intravenous vincristine or immunoglobulin.

Post-splenectomy, the platelets start to rise within 48 hours and peak at one to two weeks. The platelet count six weeks after surgery is a guide to the success of the operation, success being achieved in about 80 per cent of patients. In patients who fail to respond, steroids may be effective post-splenectomy, even where they have not helped before splenectomy.

Failure after splenectomy is a challenging problem, and the aim of treatment should be to control bleeding rather than to normalize the platelet count. Good results have been obtained with danazol, using low doses to minimize side-effects. Azathioprine (which may take many months to act) or cyclophosphamide (which acts within a few weeks) have improved patients with severe bleeding problems in up to 40 per cent of cases, but should not be prescribed without consideration of the risks of secondary malignancy.

Even temporary improvement in the platelet count may be useful to cover elective surgery or particularly bad episodes of bleeding. Vincristine (1 mg weekly) results in an improvement in the platelet count after two to three weeks in up to 70 per cent of patients, but this lasts only a few weeks. Intravenous gamma-globulin (an extremely expensive preparation, usually given as infusions of 0·4 mg/kg daily for five days) results in a rapid improvement of the platelet count in perhaps 70 per cent of patients, and this is mainly attributed to reticulo-endothelial blockade. Again, the improvement is usually short-lived, although occasional durable responses are seen.

PROGNOSIS

The prognosis of thrombocytopenia in marrow disorders depends on the underlying problem. Children with acute thrombocytopenia usually make a rapid and complete recovery, but there is a mortality of under one per cent from cerebral haemorrhage. Chronic refractory ITP has a higher mortality (although under five per cent), again mainly from cerebral haemorrhage, but the platelet count may rise with time. TTP has an extremely grave prognosis, although plasma exchange is proving to be of some value in this situation.

FURTHER READING

Karpatkin S. (1980). Review: autoimmune thrombocytopenic purpura. *Blood*, **56,** 329–343.
McMillan R. (1981). Chronic idiopathic thrombocytopenic purpura. *New Engl. J. Med.*, **304,** 1135–1147.

Chapter Nine

Pancytopenia

DEFINITION

Pancytopenia is the reduction in all cellular elements of blood, with resulting anaemia, leucopenia and thrombocytopenia.

AETIOLOGY

Pancytopenia results from reduction in marrow output or from increased destruction (*see* Table 9.1).

Severe megaloblastic change always causes anaemia but it is also a common cause of pancytopenia, which may be of such severity that patients present with bleeding from thrombyocytopenia. Less commonly, marrow output is impaired when stem cells are depleted by aplasia or by replacement of the marrow by fibrosis or secondaries from carcinomatosis. Although haematological malignancies can produce pancytopenia, the blood more often shows an increase in the cell line involved by the malignancy.

Increased destruction of cellular elements of the blood is common in the tropics from hypersplenism due to various causes; in the West, the commonest cause of hypersplenism is probably portal hypertension (*see* Chapter 12). Unexplained pancytopenia in young women raises the possibility of a diagnosis of systemic lupus erythematosus (SLE).

CLINICAL

The clinical picture reflects both the pancytopenia and the underlying cause.

Table 9.1
AETIOLOGY OF PANCYTOPENIA

Decreased production by marrow
  Stem cell reduction
    Aplasia and hypoplasia
    Paroxysmal nocturnal haemoglobinuria
  Dysplasia
    Megaloblastic anaemias
    Myelodysplasias
  Marrow replacement
    Metastases from carcinoma
    Blast cells in acute leukaemias
    Lymphoid cells in lymphomas or plasma cells in myeloma
    Fibrous tissue in myelofibrosis or bone in osteosclerosis
    Granulomata in tuberculosis

Increased destruction in the circulation
  Hypersplenism and splenomegaly
  Storage diseases
    Portal hypertension
    Haematological disorders
    Chronic infection
    Inflammation, e.g. Felty's syndrome, sarcoid
  Systemic lupus erythematosus, with immune destruction of cells
  Septicaemia (may affect marrow output too)

Details of the presentation of severe pancytopenia in aplasia are discussed in Chapter 22. Mild pancytopenia is asymptomatic and discovered only when blood is examined.

Underlying causes for pancytopenia may present in many ways. Particular note should be made of: weight loss and malaise with cough or other localizing symptoms (suggesting tuberculosis or malignancy, particularly of the bronchus, prostate, stomach and thyroid); neurological disturbances, glossitis, gastro-intestinal disease and family history (vitamin B_{12} deficiency); poor diet, which is easily overlooked in the intensive care unit (folate deficiency); lymphadenopathy, hepatosplenomegaly and skin infiltrations (haematological malignancies); and butterfly rash, pyrexia, joint problems in young women (SLE). A full drug history should not be omitted.

Table 9.2
BLOOD CHANGES THAT MAY HELP IN THE DIFFERENTIAL DIAGNOSIS IN PATIENTS WITH PANCYTOPENIA

Anaemia with
    Low reticulocytes in aplasia
    Raised reticulocytes in hypersplenism and haemolysis
    MCV > 95 fl in megaloblastic conditions, myelodysplasia and aplasia
    Teardrop-shaped cells and marked poikilocytosis in myelofibrosis
    Rouleaux formation and raised viscosity in myeloma

Leucopenia with
    Myeloblasts in acute leukaemia and myelodysplasias
    Abnormal lymphoid cells in lymphoproliferative disorders
    Plasma cells (rarely) in myeloma
    Lymphoplasmacytoid cells in macroglobulinaemia
    Hypersegmented neutrophils in megaloblastic conditions

Leuco-erythroblastic blood picture
    Carcinomatosis
    Myelofibrosis

MCV = mean corpuscular volume.

INVESTIGATIONS AND DIFFERENTIAL DIAGNOSIS

Investigation of the underlying causes of pancytopenia follows standard medical practice. Inspection of the blood film may be diagnostic, and the features of particular help are outlined in Table 9.2. The findings may lead to specific further tests, e.g. vitamin B_{12} and folate assays, serum and urine electrophoresis, antinuclear factor measurement, or Ham's test for paroxysmal nocturnal haemoglobinuria (*see* Chapter 5).

Marrow aspiration and trephine biopsy are needed to diagnose marrow infiltrations or aplasia.

TREATMENT

Treatment of the patient with cytopenias relating to the specific haematological diseases is discussed elsewhere. Where possible, treatment is also directed to the underlying cause.

Chapter Ten

Leucocytosis

The term leucocytosis is used to describe an increase in the circulating white blood cells above the normal upper limit of $11 \times 10^9/l$. The commonest reason is an increase in neutrophils, but other types of leucocytes may predominate in the differential count and give a guide to the diagnosis.

NEUTROPHILIA

Neutrophilia is an increase in neutrophil count above the normal upper limit of $7 \cdot 5 \times 10^9/l$, and this is extremely common in acute inflammation. Small increases in the neutrophil count, however, may be found in stress and after strenuous exercise, when leucocytes of normal morphology which normally line blood vessel walls are released into the free circulation. In inflammatory conditions, by contrast, the neutrophils are usually abnormal and may show toxic granulation, left shift (fewer nuclear lobes than normal), vacuolation, and even Dohle bodies. Table 10.1 shows some causes of neutrophilia.

In certain acute infections, the expected neutrophilia is not found, and this may suggest uncomplicated typhoid fever, tuberculosis, measles, mumps or varicella. Although neutrophilia is normally found in acute appendicitis and other acute inflammatory conditions, the absence of neutrophilia should not be regarded as absolute evidence against inflammation.

Myeloid Leukaemoid Reaction

A myeloid leukaemoid reaction is an extreme neutrophilia, with counts of over $50 \times 10^9/l$. This is most common in children or in

Table 10.1
CAUSES OF NEUTROPHILIA

Acute infection
  Bacterial, especially Gram-positive cocci
  Viruses, particularly in the first few days
  Spirochaetes and rickettsia

Acute inflammation
  Crohn's disease and ulcerative colitis
  Rheumatoid arthritis and polyarteritis
  Rheumatic fever
  Haemarthrosis

Necrosis
  Myocardial infarction
  Gangrene (even dry)
  Burns and crush injury
  Sickle-cell crisis

Malignancy
  Especially if there is metastasis or rapid growth

Metablic
  Diabetic ketoacidosis
  Gout
  Uraemia

Haematological
  Acute haemorrhage or haemolysis
  Proliferative disorders such as polycythaemia rubra vera

patients who have undergone splenectomy, but may be caused in others by severe forms of those diseases which normally cause a simple neutrophilia. As the name implies, the difficulty with such high counts is that they may simulate chronic granulocytic leukaemia, particularly if immature myeloid cells are released from the marrow. With leukaemoid reactions, the cause may be obvious, toxic granulation prominent, the leucocyte alkaline phosphatase (LAP) score high and chromosome analysis normal, whereas in chronic granulocytic leukaemia, the spleen is usually enlarged, the neutrophil granules normal, the LAP score low or even zero, and a Philadelphia chromosome present.

EOSINOPHILIA

Eosinophilia is said to be present when the blood eosinophil count is raised above its normal level of $0.44 \times 10^9/l$.

In the West, this most commonly reflects an allergic reaction and is found in asthma, hay fever, eczema and drug reactions. In areas where parasitic infections are endemic, hookworm, ascaris, schistosomiasis, hydatid and trichinosis are usually associated with eosinophilia, and if there is tissue invasion, high counts (over $20 \times 10^9/l$) may be found. Table 10.2 lists other causes of eosinophilia.

Table 10.2
CAUSES OF EOSINOPHILIA

Allergy
  Asthma, hay fever, angioneurotic oedema, urticaria, serum sickness
  Food and drug sensitivity, e.g. chlorpromazine

Skin disease
  Eczema, pemphigus, dermatitis herpetiformis, psoriasis

Parasitic infections
  Especially of intestine or with tissue involvement

Neoplasia
  Particularly Hodgkin's disease, and tumours with metastases or necrosis

Haematological
  Polycythaemia rubra vera, chronic granulocytic leukaemia, and others
  Eosinophilic leukaemia (*see* text)

Immunological
  Wiskott–Aldrich syndrome
  Hyper-IgE with infections
  Selective IgA deficiency

Miscellaneous
  Polyarteritis nodosa, rheumatoid and systemic lupus
  Sarcoid, post-splenectomy
  Hypereosinophilic syndrome—no parasite demonstrable
  Drug reactions
  Loeffler's syndrome
  Tropical eosinophilia

Diagnosis

In most cases, the diagnosis is clear from the history. Where there is a story suggesting an allergic disorder, skin tests may be positive, IgE levels may be raised, and IgE antibodies to appropriate antigens may be demonstrable by radio-immunoabsorbent tests (RAST). In patients where parasitic infection is likely, fresh faecal specimens for ova and parasites are helpful. Duodenal aspiration is used in diagnosis of strongyloidiasis.

Loeffler's Pneumonia

Loeffler's pneumonia (also known as Loeffler's syndrome) is a term applied to a marked blood eosinophilia associated with transitory and patchy pulmonary infiltrates, caused by an allergic reaction of the host to migration of parasitic larvae through the lungs. Eosinophils may be abundant in the sputum.

Hypereosinophilic Syndrome

Loeffler also described a serious endocarditis associated with eosinophilia, which would now be categorized under the term hypereosinophilic syndrome (HES). By definition, there is an eosinophilia of $> 1500 \times 10^9/l$ persisting for over six months, with no evidence of any other known cause of eosinophilia on careful investigation and with symptoms and signs of HES organ involvement which can be attributed to the eosinophilia. The syndrome is distinct but undoubtedly comprises a heterogeneous group of disorders. The patient is generally unwell with weight loss and fever.

The progressive organ damage seen in HES is believed to be secondary to tissue infiltration with eosinophils, damage related to eosinophil products, or thrombo-embolic phenomena from thrombi associated with endocardial damage. Such organ damage is occasionally seen in other patients with severe eosinophilia of known cause.

The organs affected include skin (rashes, dermatographia and angio-oedema), heart (endocardial fibrosis with valvular incompetence, heart failure and sometimes overlying thrombus with multiple emboli), lung (with progressive inflammation, effusions and fibrosis), liver (hepatomegaly), gut (diarrhoea, nausea and cramps) and eye (usually embolic problems).

The syndrome may occur at any age, but is most common between 20 and 50 years old. The median survival without treatment is under one year, but vigorous supportive treatment, supplemented by steroids if there is evidence of progression (and, if needed, hydroxyurea aimed at keeping the leucocyte count under $10\,000 \times 10^9/l$), has improved survival and quality of life very considerably. If the eosinophil count is $> 100\,000 \times 10^9/l$, leucopheresis has been used on a temporary basis.

Eosinophilic Leukaemia

Eosinophilic leukaemia is a term which has been used to describe a rare disorder with a very high eosinophil count (in the absence of any known cause) with immature and abnormal forms in the blood (hypogranulation and vacuoles), anaemia, thrombocytopenia and eosinophilic hyperplasia in the marrow with cytogenetic abnormalities. However, all these abnormalities have been described as part of HES, and it may be that, at least on occasions, HES is caused by a primary haematological problem.

LYMPHOCYTOSIS

In lymphocytosis, the blood lymphocyte count is raised above the normal limit ($3.5 \times 10^9/l$ in adults and $8.5 \times 10^9/l$ in children). It is common in viral infections but may also be found with tuberculosis, brucellosis or syphilis.

Reactive lymphocytosis with very high counts (above $25 \times 10^9/l$) is sometimes referred to as a lymphocytic leukaemoid reaction. It may be found in whooping cough and in infectious lymphocytosis, an uncommon disease occurring in small epidemics in children, perhaps caused by an enterovirus. High counts in middle-aged and elderly people are usually due to chronic lymphocytic leukaemia.

Atypical mononuclear cells associated with a lymphocytosis are classically found in infectious mononucleosis (IM) in teenagers, but may also be seen in hepatitis and in cytomegalovirus and toxoplasma infections. Where the diagnosis is in doubt, tests for the IM heterophil antibody and tests to show rising titres of virus antibody are usually of help.

MONOCYTOSIS

A blood monocyte count above the normal upper limit of $0.8 \times 10^9/l$ is termed monocytosis. This is most commonly found in chronic infections, where it can be helpful in pointing the investigations towards excluding tuberculosis, subacute bacterial endocarditis and brucellosis, which may all present with obscure fever and malaise. In older patients who are well, evidence of chronic myelomonocytic leukaemia should be sought (lymphadenopathy, splenomegaly and abnormal monocyte morphology, *see* Chapter 20). Monocytosis in some countries may suggest protozoal or rickettsial infection. Other causes of a monocytosis are included in Table 10.3.

BASOPHILIA

Basophils contain heparin, histamine and chemotactic factors and, together with tissue mast cells, are important in immediate hypersensitivity reactions. They are present in such small numbers in the blood that the percentage quoted in repeated manual differential counts on 100 cells on the same normal blood

Table 10.3
CAUSES OF MONOCYTOSIS

Chronic infection
  Bacterial: Subacute bacterial endocarditis, tuberculosis, brucellosis
  Protozoal: Malaria, leishmaniasis
  Rickettsial: Typhus, Rocky Mountain spotted fever

Malignancy
  Hodgkin's disease and occasionally in carcinomatosis

Haematological
  Chronic myelomonocytic leukaemia
  Acute monocytic leukaemia
  In myeloproliferative disorders, such as polycythaemia rubra vera
  Marrow recovery after cytotoxic therapy

film may vary from zero to four per cent for purely statistical reasons. Even when they can be counted accurately, they do not show helpful changes in allergic reactions. A persistent increase above $0.1 \times 10^9/l$ is found in chronic granulocytic leukaemia, but this increase is usually dwarfed by the increase in neutrophils and myelocytes. An increase may be seen in other myeloproliferative disorders, and also in pox infections.

FURTHER READING

Klebanoff S. J., Clark R. A. (1978). *The Neutrophil: Function and Clinical Disorders.* Oxford: North-Holland Publishing Company.

Chapter Eleven

Thrombocytosis

DEFINITION

Thrombocytosis is an increase in peripheral blood platelet concentration (normal range 150–400 × 10^9/l).

The introduction of routine automated platelet counting has led to the recognition that thrombocytosis may accompany many medical and surgical disorders (*see* Table 11.1).

BACKGROUND AND PATHOLOGY

Most patients with a platelet count between 500 and 1000 × 10^9/l will have a secondary or 'reactive' thrombocytosis. Above 1000 × 10^9/l, the probability of primary (essential) thrombocythaemia increases with the degree of thrombocytosis. Chronic bleeding may cause thrombocytosis, as erythropoietin may stimulate both red cell and platelet production. Primary thrombocythaemia is a malignant disorder which belongs to the spectrum of myeloproliferative disorders (including polycythaemia vera and primary myelofibrosis).

SYMPTOMS AND SIGNS

Patients with reactive thrombocytosis (*see* Table 11.1) exhibit the clinical features of the underlying disease. In the absence of an obvious cause, a particular effort should be made to exclude occult gastro-intestinal bleeding and/or neoplasia. A raised platelet count per se is rarely directly associated with thrombotic problems in this situation (other factors such as venous stasis and trauma in surgical patients, or a 'procoagulant' diathesis in

Table 11.1
CAUSES OF THROMBOCYTOSIS

Primary haematological disorders
  Primary (essential) thrombocythaemia
  Other myeloproliferative disorders
  Chronic granulocytic leukaemia
  Associated with myelodysplasia (especially $5q^-$ karyotype)

Secondary (reactive)
  Haemorrhage (especially gastro-intestinal bleeding)
  Iron deficiency
  Malignancy (e.g. gastro-intestinal, breast and lung, Hodgkin's disease)
  Inflammatory bowel disease (Crohn's disease, ulcerative colitis)
  Post-splenectomy
  After surgery or trauma
  Infection (including tuberculosis)
  Rheumatoid disease
  Exercise

cancer patients, are more relevant). Thrombocytosis after splenectomy is usually transient (peaking at two to three weeks) but may be associated with an increased risk of thrombosis and pulmonary embolism in the post-operative period.

Primary thrombocythaemia is largely a disease of the middle-aged and elderly. Its clinical features may include the systemic symptoms, such as pruritis and sweating, characteristic of other myeloproliferative disorders. Haemorrhage, especially gastro-intestinal, post-surgical and spontaneous bruising, tends to dominate the clinical picture, and qualitative defects of platelet function are found. Thrombotic events may occur in the same patient, the spectrum ranging from calf vein or cerebral thrombosis to thrombosis of the hepatic or splenic veins. A minority of patients present with a distinctive syndrome of painful digital ischaemia and acrocyanosis. There is also an increased incidence of peptic disease.

About 40 per cent of patients with primary thrombocythaemia have moderate splenomegaly, although splenic atrophy may develop in the course of the disease. Hepatomegaly is less common (16 per cent).

INVESTIGATIONS AND DIFFERENTIAL DIAGNOSIS

The aim of investigation is to distinguish primary thrombocythaemia from the many secondary causes. This is often achieved by a process of exclusion. Special investigations will depend on the clinical context but will often include endoscopic and radiological techniques to exclude gastro-intestinal haemorrhage, inflammation or malignancy. Presence of splenomegaly (demonstrated by ultrasound or isotope scan) favours primary thrombocythaemia. Thrombocytosis in chronic granulocytic leukaemia or myelodysplasia would be diagnosed by the characteristic clinical and haematological picture (*see* Chapters 16 and 20).

In primary thrombocythaemia, the platelet count is usually greater than $1000 \times 10^9/l$ at diagnosis. Features of generalized myeloproliferation, such as leucocytosis and mild polycythaemia, may be seen and cases may progress to polycythaemia vera or myelofibrosis. Chronic bleeding is associated with a hypochromic microcytic red cell picture, and the presence of Howell–Jolly bodies implies that splenic atrophy has occurred. Neutrophil alkaline phosphatase is often increased but is of little diagnostic value. Although standard coagulation tests are normal, the bleeding time is often prolonged and in vitro platelet function tests are abnormal. Bone marrow trephine biopsy is more useful in diagnosis than aspiration alone. Typical features include increased cellularity and megakaryocytes, often with an increase in other myeloid and erythroid elements (panmyelosis), and an increase in reticulin fibres. The increased haemopoietic activity may cause hyperuricaemia and folate depletion (much more common in polycythaemia vera or myelofibrosis). There is wide variation in disease activity between individual patients, ranging from a static, mild thrombocytosis to a rapidly progressive myeloproliferative disorder.

TREATMENT

Reactive thrombocytosis may respond to treatment of the underlying disease. Monitoring platelet count can be a useful index of disease activity and response to treatment in inflammatory bowel disease. Transient thrombocytosis after splenectomy is common. The true risk of thrombotic events is uncertain, as is the value of prophylactic aspirin or heparin in this context.

In primary thrombocythaemia, the risk of both haemorrhagic and thrombotic complications is reduced by normalization of the platelet count. It is conventional to administer either intravenous radiophosphorus (^{32}P, a β-emitter) or an oral alkylating agent such as busulphan. Both may reduce the platelet count over a few weeks. ^{32}P may produce sustained remissions (3–12 months) and is convenient for administration to the elderly. Busulphan carries a higher risk of unpredictable and dangerously prolonged pancytopenia. Both ^{32}P and alkylating agents are leukaemogenic (*see* Chapter 19), and their administration to younger patients is problematical. The oral antimetabolite, hydroxyurea, may produce a rapid effect and is probably non-leukaemogenic. However, it has a short duration of action and daily administration is usually required. Nevertheless, hydroxyurea should be considered in the younger patient. If an extremely rapid reduction in platelet count is desired, intensive platelet pheresis using an automated cell-separator may be useful until myelosuppressive treatment is effective. The use of aspirin to prevent thrombotic complications in primary thrombocythaemia produces an unacceptable incidence of serious bleeding which outweighs any benefit (Murphy *et al.*, 1986), and aspirin-like drugs should also be avoided. However, short-term administration of low-dose aspirin may be dramatically effective in the subgroup presenting with acrocyanosis and digital ischaemia. Allopurinol may be a useful adjunctive treatment if hyperuricaemia is present. There is recent evidence that α-interferon may be used successfully to control the platelet count in primary thrombocythaemia.

PROGNOSIS

The prognosis of reactive thrombocytosis depends on the underlying disease.

Reported median survival for primary thrombocythaemia varies widely, but is probably in the region of 10 years. Early deaths are generally due to bleeding or thrombosis. Later in the course, there may be transition towards more generalized myeloproliferation or myelofibrosis, and secondary leukaemias start to appear about five years after myelosuppressive therapy is initiated.

FURTHER READING

Murphy S., Lland H., Rosenthal D., Laszlo J. (1986). Essential thrombocythaemia: an interim report from the Polycythaemia Vera Study Group. *Semin. Hematol.*, **23**, 177–182.

Chapter Twelve

Disorders of the Spleen

SPLENOMEGALY

Definition

A palpable spleen usually implies underlying disease. Radiological techniques show that the spleen has already enlarged to twice its normal size (150 g in an adult) before it becomes palpable. Owing to anatomical variations, a spleen of normal volume may occasionally be palpable, particularly in infancy.

Aetiology

Splenomegaly may be the result of a wide range of pathological processes, including haematological problems, infection, inflammation, infiltration and congestion (*see* Table 12.1).

The commonest causes of splenomegaly vary considerably from one country to another. In the West, haematological proliferative diseases and portal hypertension are important. In tropical regions, splenomegaly is very common (over half of hospital in-patients have splenomegaly), and although portal hypertension remains important, parasitic infections with malaria, leishmaniasis and schistosomiasis predominate. Idiopathic splenomegaly (tropical splenomegaly) is common in New Guinea and Central America. Travellers from the West visiting tropical countries have poor immunity to malaria, and prophylactic drugs are frequently not taken for a sufficient time (four weeks) after return.

Splenomegaly is common in young Negro children with sickle-cell disease, but it should be remembered that by the age of about 10 years, repeated splenic infarction has usually rendered the

Table 12.1
CLASSIFICATION OF CAUSES OF SPLENOMEGALY

Haematological
  Proliferations
    Red cell — Polycythaemia rubra vera
    Myeloid — Chronic granulocytic leukaemia
              Myelofibrosis
              Myelodysplasias
              Acute myeloid leukaemia (minimal enlargement, if any)
    Lymphoid — Chronic lymphocytic leukaemia
               Hodgkin's disease and non-Hodgkin's lymphoma
               Prolymphocytic leukaemia and hairy-cell leukaemia
    Plasma cell — Myeloma (10% of cases only) and immunocytomas
    Platelet — Primary thrombocythaemia
  Haemolytic anaemias — Thalassaemia and many others
  Deficiency anaemias — Iron deficiency and megaloblastic (only slight enlargement)

Infections
  Bacterial — Septicaemia and subacute bacterial endocarditis
              Tuberculosis and brucellosis
  Virus — Glandular fever and others
  Tropical — Malaria, leishmaniasis, schistosomiasis

Inflammations
  Tropical splenomegaly
  Sarcoid
  Rheumatoid arthritis and systemic lupus erythematosus

Congestion
  Cirrhosis with portal hypertension
  Splenic vein occlusion

Infiltrations
  Amyloid
  Storage disorders (e.g. lipid storage diseases, mucopolysaccharidoses)

Non-haematological proliferations
  Polycystic disease
  Hamartomas
  Metastatic tumour (surprisingly rare)

spleen impalpable. Thalassaemia is widespread but particularly common in the Mediterranean, Middle East, India, and Far East.

Storage diseases, many of which are recessively inherited, are found particularly where there is consanguinity.

Symptoms

Patients with splenomegaly exhibit the clinical features of the underlying diseases, and clinical enquiry is directed to this end, bearing in mind the geographical situation. A travel history is an essential part of clinical evaluation.

Direct enquiry may elicit a story of past umbilical sepsis (portal vein thrombosis), trauma (haematoma), rheumatic fever with recent malaise and fever, (subacute bacterial endocarditis), jaundice or alcohol ingestion (portal hypertension).

A history relating directly to the problem in the spleen is sometimes obtained. Pain over the spleen or left shoulder (from diaphragmatic irritation) is typical of splenic infarction, a common presentation of chronic granulocytic leukaemia (CGL), myeloproliferative syndromes and sickle-cell disease. A feeling of fullness after eating only moderately sized meals is often found where splenic enlargement is considerable.

Signs

An enlarged spleen must be distinguished from other masses in the left upper quadrant, notably the left kidney, tumours of the splenic flexure of the colon or stomach, and retroperitoneal masses. Classically, the spleen moves downwards and medially with respiration, is smooth (apart from a medial notch), and is dull to percussion (which may extend to the left base of the chest laterally and posteriorly). By contrast with most enlarged kidneys, the spleen is not normally ballotable and its upper border cannot be palpated because it is above the ribs. Occasionally, a splenic rub with respiration may be heard when the spleen surface is inflamed, particularly after painful infarcts. An arterial bruit, reflecting increased blood flow to a greatly enlarged spleen, can occasionally be heard.

The size of the spleen may be helpful in diagnosis. In the West, a very large spleen with its lower margin below the umbilicus is common in CGL and myelofibrosis, and is also found in some rare diseases (e.g. prolymphocytic leukaemia, hairy-cell leukaemia, storage diseases). In sandfly areas, visceral leishmaniasis may present with huge splenomegaly, wasting and pigmentation of the skin (giving rise to the name kala-azar). In these conditions, the splenomegaly tends to dominate the abdominal findings, but there may be some hepatomegaly. Lymphadenopathy is usually absent or minimal, which contrasts with the findings in lymphoma. Splenomegaly is usually fairly slight in SBE, non-tropical infections, collagen diseases, deficiency anaemias and thyrotoxicosis.

Anaemia is common and reflects the underlying conditions. In association with jaundice, it suggests a haemolytic disease or liver disease. In association with lymphadenopathy or hepatomegaly, it suggests a haematological proliferative disease.

A pyrexia may have an obvious cause such as malaria, but pyrexia of unknown origin should lead to a search for splinter haemorrhages, changing cardiac murmurs (and abnormal echo cardiography), fundal haemorrhages, microscopic haematuria and repeated blood cultures, in an attempt to diagnose SBE. Antibody studies may be helpful in the diagnosis of brucella and other infections.

Investigations

The history and signs guide the intelligent choice of investigations in patients with splenomegaly. A full blood count and liver function tests usually narrow the diagnostic spectrum, and the blood film appearance dictates appropriate investigations for haemolysis. Marrow aspiration and trephine biopsy often clinch the diagnosis of haematological disorders.

Where infection is suspected, standard microbiological tests are needed. Radiography of the chest may reveal the lung and node abnormalities of tuberculosis, sarcoid or lymphoma.

A plain abdominal X-ray is sometimes needed to confirm that the enlarged organ is spleen. The exact size and the presence of internal tumours and cysts of the spleen can be shown by ultrasound studies, computerized tomography scans, and liver and spleen scans (using technetium or chromium-labelled heat-damaged red cells), which may also reveal other abdominal abnormalities.

There are sophisticated methods available using radioactive markers and counters to delineate splenic blood flow, splenic red cell and plasma pool size, red cell survival and red cell and platelet destruction in the spleen, splenic haemopoiesis and the presence of accessory spleens. On occasion, a laparotomy with splenectomy is needed for diagnosis.

Treatment

The treatment of splenomegaly is usually the treatment of the underlying disease. Local treatment, in the form of splenectomy, radiotherapy or arterial embolization, are indicated in a few conditions.

Splenectomy

Splenectomy is usually indicated in traumatic rupture of the spleen. It is normally the treatment of choice in hereditary spherocytosis and can be curative in idiopathic thrombocytopenia resistant to steroids. It may be helpful in patients with portal hypertension, and in some patients with hypersplenism the blood counts may rise sufficiently to improve the clinical problems. With isolated and unexplained splenomegaly, splenectomy may be justified to make a diagnosis, and a lymphoma may be discovered by this means. The vogue for carrying out a staging laparotomy in established Hodgkin's disease has passed. Although treatment with interferon has greatly improved the outlook for patients with hairy-cell leukaemia, splenectomy remains helpful in patients with considerable splenomegaly.

Early postoperative complications include local haemorrhage, which may lead to a subphrenic abscess, thrombo-embolic problems and respiratory infection. Good haemostasis at operation, breathing exercises and early mobilization are important in the prevention of these problems. Some authors advocate aspirin therapy (75 mg daily) when the platelet count is above $600 \times 10^9/l$ during the reactive thrombocytopenia, which is usually seen at 7–14 days post-splenectomy.

Later problems are predominantly those of infection. Destruction of the spleen by any process renders the patient more vulnerable to any pyogenic infection, notably with encapsulated organisms such as meningococcus and pneumococcus, which may be life-threatening. Listeria infection may occur at any age and, in appropriate areas, malaria may flare up. The problems are particularly severe in young children, and so splenectomy is generally avoided at this age. Pneumococcal vaccination before splenectomy and life-long oral penicillin prophylaxis after splenectomy have been shown to be helpful.

The prognosis of patients after splenectomy reflects their underlying disease. In uncomplicated hereditary spherocytosis, for example, the mortality in experienced hands is very low, whereas in advanced malignancy in the elderly, it is considerable.

Other

Radiotherapy to the spleen has been used with good effect on its own for chronic lymphocytic leukaemia, even where the spleen is not particularly enlarged. With lymphomas, radiotherapy to the spleen is usually combined with radiotherapy to nodal areas, and often in combination with chemotherapy.

Where surgery is contra-indicated, arterial embolization has been used with success, but there are complications, which include embolization of the wrong organ (e.g. liver), abscess formation and disseminated intravascular coagulation.

HYPERSPLENISM

Definition

Hypersplenism is enlargement of the spleen with premature removal of blood cells causing reduction of one or more types of blood cells (red cells, leucocytes and platelets) despite normal marrow production. Confirmation of the diagnosis is made only if the condition is corrected by splenectomy.

Clinical

The spleen is moderately or considerably enlarged, and the findings are those of the underlying condition. The anaemia is usually moderate (8–10 g/dl) with red cells of mainly normal appearance. Thrombocytopenia is usually slight, but there may be severe neutropenia with recurrent infections.

Treatment

In addition to treatment of the underlying disease, splenectomy may be warranted to reduce problems of recurrent infections or high transfusion requirements.

HYPOSPLENISM

Hyposplenism is a diagnosis made from the blood film appearance, and it has both clinical and diagnostic importance.

Clinical

The blood signs of hyposplenism are found after splenectomy (unless splenunculae have grown to replace the spleen function) and after multiple infarction, such as is found in primary thrombocythaemia or in older children with sickle-cell disease. Hyposplenism is also seen in coeliac disease, Crohn's disease, ulcerative colitis and dermatitis herpetiformis, where careful scrutiny of the blood film may provide the first clue to the diagnosis. It is interesting to note that the splenic atrophy seen in coeliac disease is not usually corrected by a gluten-free diet.

Investigation

The blood shows a normal haemoglobin, but the red cells are abnormal with target cells, irregular contracted cells, Howell–Jolly bodies (nuclear remnants) and, sometimes, siderotic granules. There may be a persistent increase in monocytes and lymphocytes. After splenectomy, the platelet count peaks (usually under $1000 \times 10^9/1$) in the second week and then usually returns to normal within about two months, unless there is persistent anaemia.

Treatment

The prevention of infections after splenectomy has been mentioned above, and is relevant to other causes of hyposplenism.

FURTHER READING

Bowdler A.J. (1983). Splenomegaly and hypersplenism. *Clinics in Haematology*, **12**(2), 467–412.

Richards J.D.M. (1976). Hypersplenism. *Br. J. Hosp. Med.*, **15**, 405–412.

Chapter Thirteen

Bleeding Problems

PHYSIOLOGY OF HAEMOSTASIS

The principle function of haemostasis is to arrest bleeding from damaged blood vessels. There are two major components – platelets and coagulation factors. Platelets normally circulate close to the endothelial surface and thus are in close proximity to damaged endothelial cells and subendothelial structures when trauma to the endothelial surface occurs. Many coagulation factors circulate as pro-enzymes, which are converted into active proteolytic enzymes following a suitable stimulus. A cascading event (Fig. 13.1 and 3) then follows with activation of other coagulation factors. This is an amplification process, the end result being the formation of fibrin. For normal haemostasis to occur, adequate numbers of functioning platelets and coagulation factors must therefore be present.

When bleeding occurs, both platelets and coagulation factors are exposed to subendothelial structures, in particular to collagen. This produces a sequence of membrane and biochemical changes within platelets, which act to increase the total surface area of platelets, to make their membranes sticky and to cause the release of a variety of substances from within platelet cytoplasmic granules, especially ADP, which accentuates the above mentioned changes. The net result of this is that platelets adhere to collagen and aggregate to each other, producing a 'platelet plug' which is responsible for the initial cessation of bleeding.

The coagulation cascade is artificially divided, based on the common laboratory screening tests (Fig. 13.1), into the intrinsic and extrinsic systems. Activation of the intrinsic system results in the formation of activated factor XII (XIIa). The extrinsic system requires the activation of factor VII (VIIa) which follows the interaction between factor VII and tissue factor, a phospho-

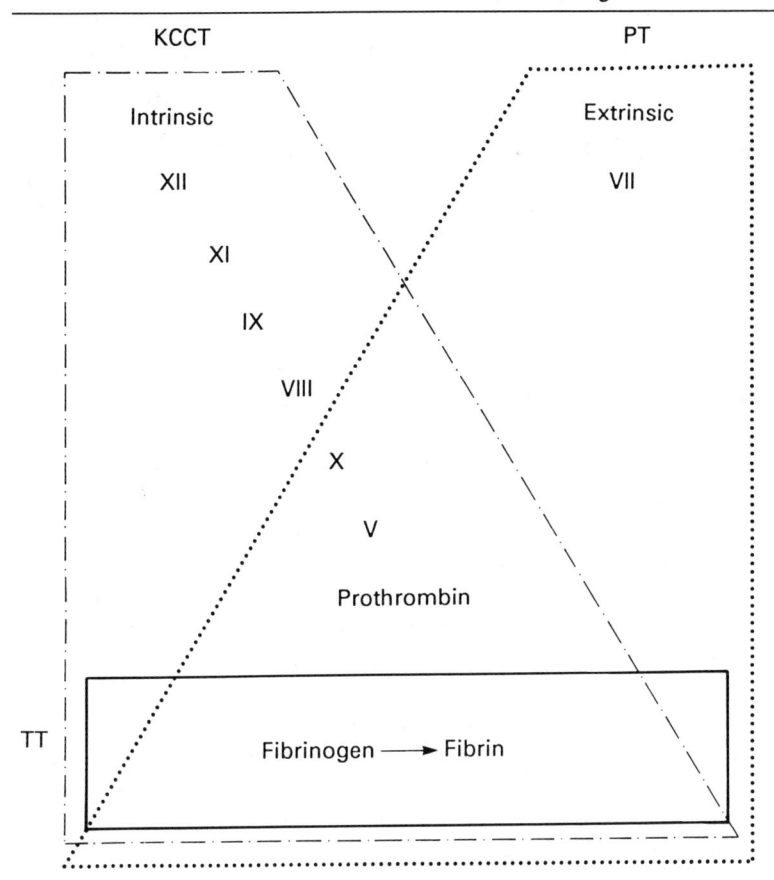

Fig. 13.1. Aspects of the coagulation cascade measured by the kaolin cephalin clotting time (KCCT), prothrombin time (PT) and thrombin time (TT).

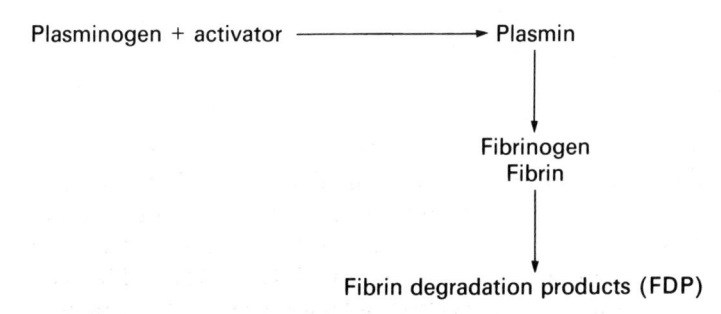

Plasminogen + activator ⟶ Plasmin
                                    ↓
                              Fibrinogen
                              Fibrin
                                    ↓
                    Fibrin degradation products (FDP)

Fig. 13.2. Fibrinolysis

lipid released by damaged endothelial cells. The intrinsic and extrinsic systems do not work independently in vivo, as a number of links promoting cross activation between them have been demonstrated. From this complex biochemical sequence of events, an insoluble protein, fibrin, is formed, which then adheres to the platelet plug. Without the formation of fibrin, the platelet aggregates formed may eventually be 'washed' away, with the commencement of bleeding again. Most coagulation factors are formed in the liver. Vitamin K is necessary for the biological activity of prothrombin (II) and factors VII, IX and X. Factor VIII von Willebrand factor (a deficiency of which causes von Willebrand's disease) is produced by vascular endothelial cells. The site of synthesis of factor VIII coagulant protein (a deficiency of which causes haemophilia) is the liver, although the exact cell of origin is unknown.

Following the cessation of bleeding, the platelet–fibrin plug is eventually removed by the fibrinolytic system (Fig. 13.2). This depends on the release of plasminogen activator from damaged vascular endothelial cells. Plasminogen activator and circulating plasminogen (an inactive pro-enzyme) then adhere to newly formed fibrin. From plasminogen, plasmin is formed. This potent proteolytic enzyme is capable of degrading a number of coagulation proteins, in particular fibrinogen and fibrin. These large molecular weight proteins are then broken down into smaller units (fibrin degradation products, FDP) which are readily removed by the cells of the reticulo-endothelial system. FDP are not simply inert end products, but possess anticoagulant properties capable of inhibiting thrombin activity and thus further fibrin formation.

TESTS OF PLATELET ACTIVITY

Platelet Count

A platelet count is performed to exclude thrombocytopenia.

Intrinsic system

XII ⟶ XIIa

XI ⟶ XIa

IX ⟶ IXa

           VIII

X ⟶ Xa

Extrinsic system

VII ⟶ VIIa

        VA

Prothrombin (II) ⟶ Thrombin

Fibrinogen (I) ⟶ Fibrin

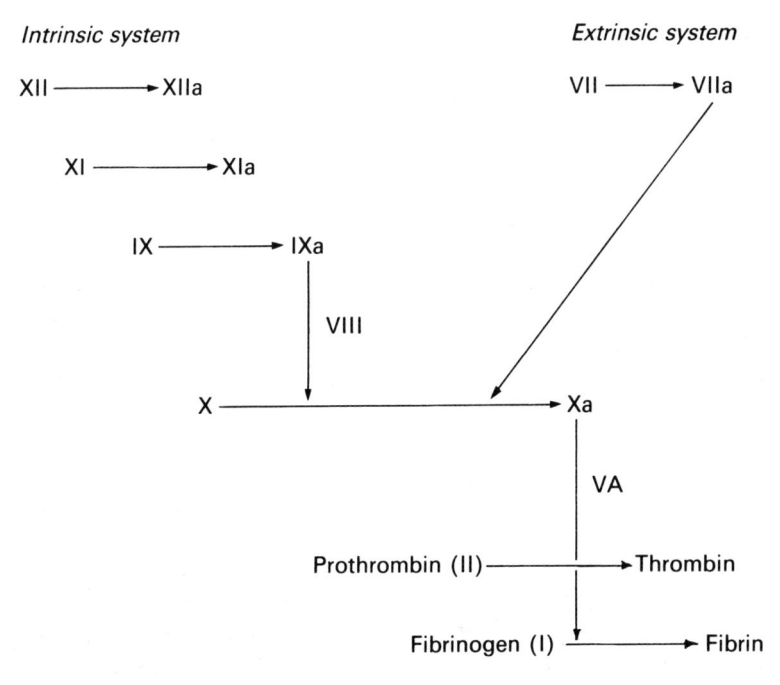

Fig. 13.3. The coagulative cascade.

Bleeding Time

A bleeding time is performed on the skin of the forearm using a template which allows a longitudinal incision of known length and depth to be made. Variants, such as blood flow through the limb, are standardized by using a sphygmomanometer inflated to 40 mmHg around the upper arm. Normally, following an incision, bleeding stops within nine minutes. A prolonged bleeding time together with a normal platelet count suggests the presence of dysfunctional platelets. In this situation, more specific tests of platelet function may be indicated, looking for defects of platelet membrane glycoproteins, prostaglandin metabolism or abnormalities of intracytoplasmic platelet granules. In most patients who have dysfunctional platelets, a simple screening test, such as in vitro platelet aggregation in response to such agents as ADP, collagen and adrenaline, is abnormal.

TESTS OF COAGULATION FUNCTION see fig. 13.1

The differential diagnosis of bleeding disorders based on abnormalities of KCCT, PT and TT is shown in Table 13.1.

Kaolin Cephalin Clotting Time (KCCT) and Activated Partial Thromboplastin Time (APTT)

These parameters measure the activity of the intrinsic system of the coagulation cascade. A normal KCCT will therefore require adequate amounts of functioning factors XII, XI, IX, VIII, X, V, prothrombin and fibrinogen.

Prothrombin Time (PT)

This measures the activity of the extrinsic system of the coagulation cascade. A normal PT requires adequate amounts of functioning factors VII, X, V, prothrombin and fibrinogen.

Thrombin Time (TT)

Thrombin time measures the formation of fibrin from fibrinogen. This is the final phase of the coagulation cascade, and therefore a prolonged TT is usually accompanied by prolongation of PT and KCCT.

Specific Coagulation Factor Assays

These can identify a deficiency of a coagulation factor which may occur secondary to reduced production or increased consumption. Very rarely, coagulation factor deficiencies may occur on an immune basis.

TESTS OF FIBRINOLYTIC ACTIVITY

As plasmin causes degradation of fibrin, fibrinogen and other coagulation factors, excess plasmin activity may be accompanied by:

1. Low circulating fibrinogen levels
2. Raised FDP levels
3. A prolonged thrombin time.

If excessive fibrinolysis is suspected, further more specific tests, such as an euglobulin clot lysis time and the measurement of circulating plasmin and plasminogen levels, may be indicated.

CONGENITAL DISORDERS OF HAEMOSTASIS

Platelet Disorders

These include membrane abnormalities, intracellular abnormalities and enzyme deficiencies. The clinical manifestations vary between a subclinical disorder with no bleeding manifestations to a serious haemorrhagic disorder such as thrombasthenia.

Table 13.1
DIAGNOSTIC GUIDE TO ABNORMALITIES OF KCCT, PT AND TT

Test	N or P	Differential diagnosis
KCCT	P	Haemophilia
PT	N	Christmas disease
TT	N	Von Willebrand's disease
		Inhibitors of factors XII, XI, IX or VIII
		Lupus inhibitor
KCCT	P	Warfarin therapy
PT	P	Massive transfusion syndrome
TT	N	Vitamin K deficiency
		Factors X, V or II deficiency
KCCT	P	Heparin therapy
PT	P	DIC
TT	P	Hypofibrinogenaemia
		Dysfibrinogenaemia

KCCT = kaolin cephalin clotting time; PT = prothrombin time; TT = thrombin time; DIC = disseminated intravascular coagulation; N = normal; P = prolonged.

Membrane abnormalities

The Bernard–Soulier (giant platelet) syndrome is characterized by the presence of large platelets, thrombocytopenia and abnormal in vitro platelet aggregation tests. The membrane defect has been characterized as a deficiency of glycoprotein 1b and is inherited in an autosomal fashion. A mild to moderate bleeding disorder follows the lack of adherence of platelets to subendothelial collagen. Glanzmann's thrombasthenia is a severe bleeding disorder associated with a lack of platelet membrane glycoprotein IIb/IIIa. It is also inherited in an autosomal fashion. In vitro platelet aggregation to ADP, collagen and adrenaline is virtually absent, and unlike the Bernard–Soulier syndrome, platelet numbers and morphology are normal.

Intracellular defects

A variety of defects may occur, characterized by either a deficiency of intraplatelet dense granules (which contain ADP and serotonin) or an inability to release ADP from such granules, resulting in a mild bleeding disorder. Easy bruising or prolonged oozing after surgery or trauma may occur. These syndromes are recognized in the laboratory by abnormal platelet aggregation studies. Electron microscopy may be useful when a reduction in dense granule numbers is suspected.

Enzyme deficiencies

Normal platelet function depends on the intracellular formation of prostaglandins by activated platelets (Fig. 13.4). Specific enzyme deficiencies, e.g. cyclo-oxygenase and thromboxane synthetase deficiencies, are associated with a mild bleeding disorder. Abnormal in vitro platelet aggregation studies may suggest such a defect.

Coagulation Factor Disorders

Haemophilia and Christmas disease

These are both sex-linked recessive disorders, the abnormal gene being carried on the X chromosome. Therefore, males inherit the disease while the carrier state is confined to females, who also

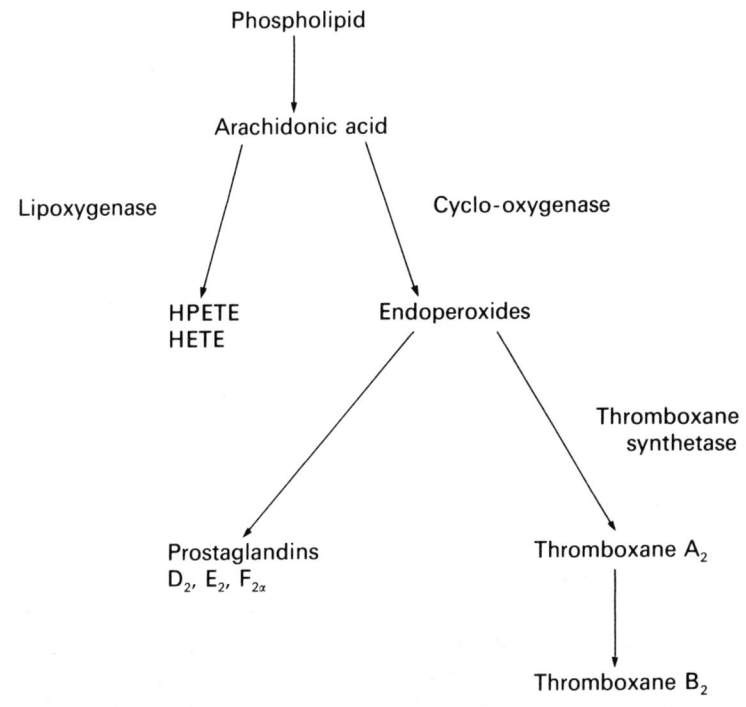

Fig. 13.4. Prostaglandin metabolism in platelets. HPETE=12-hydroperoxyeicosatetraenoic acid. HETE=12-hydroxyeicosatetraenoic acid.

have a normal X chromosome (Fig. 13.5). Rarely, the disease may occur in females when both X chromosomes are affected. Haemophilia is due to a deficiency of factor VIII coagulant protein, and Christmas disease is due to a lack of factor IX. Clinically, the diseases are indistinguishable, and laboratory assays of factors VIII and IX are necessary for a specific diagnosis.

Problems usually first occur in the second year of life. Recurrent spontaneous non-traumatic haemarthroses affecting the large hinge joints of the knees and elbows is a classical feature of these diseases. Other joints, particularly the ankles, may be affected, but it is unusual for bleeding to occur into the small joints of the hands and feet. Repeated bleeding episodes over many years result in progressive deterioration and destruction of the joint with impaired movement, flexion contractures and associated muscle wasting and weakness. Bleeding may also occur into

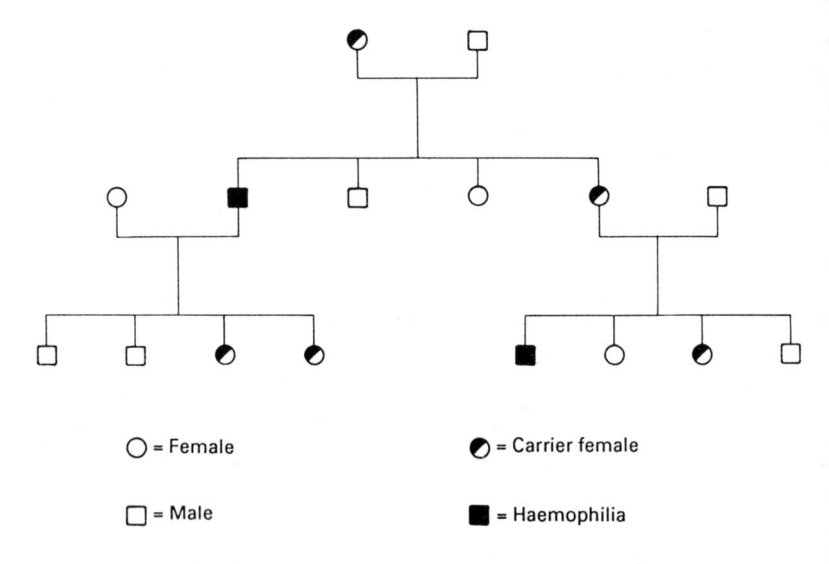

Fig. 13.5. Inheritance pattern of haemophilia.

○ = Female
□ = Male
◐ = Carrier female
■ = Haemophilia

muscles, and a characteristic presentation is that of an iliopsoas muscle bleed, with involvement of the lateral cutaneous nerve of thigh, producing sensory loss over the anterior aspect of the thigh. Occasionally, muscle or subperiosteal bleeds may not resolve and evolve into progressively enlarging haematomas (pseudotumours).

The severity of these disorders depends directly on the baseline coagulation factor levels. Spontaneous bleeding is rare when factor VIII or IX levels are greater then 0·05 U/ml (normal range 0·5–2·0 U/ml). These patients may, however, experience prolonged post-traumatic or post-surgical bleeding. Severe disease (levels less than 0·02 U/ml) results in repeated spontaneous bleeding episodes.

Approximately six per cent of haemophiliacs and less than one per cent of Christmas disease patients develop antibodies to factor VIII and IX. This usually occurs in the late teens after many years of treatment. The reason why this phenomenon should occur in some patients is not known.

Treatment of these diseases involves a multidisciplinary approach involving haematologists, physiotherapists, orthopaedic surgeons, social workers and dentists in particular. The main stem of treatment is an intravenous infusion of factor-specific concentrate when a bleeding episode occurs, which may be two to three times per week in severely affected patients. The development of home-based therapy is an important milestone in haemophilia care. Patients are taught a venepuncture technique and can therefore treat themselves at home, avoiding the delay which occurs with hospital treatment.

The side effects of treatment are:

1. *Allergic reactions* These occur infrequently and usually resolve by changing to a different factor concentrate 'brand'.
2. *Hepatitis* Factor concentrates expose patients to plasma pooled from many thousands of blood donors. In recent years, the careful screening of donors for hepatitis-B has greatly decreased the transfer of this virus, but there is no useful test for the non-A, non-B viruses. The majority, if not all, of multi-infused patients have therefore been exposed to the non-A, non-B hepatitis virus or viruses. While acute hepatitis with jaundice and constitutional upset occurs infrequently, about 70 per cent of patients consistently have abnormal liver function tests with raised transaminase levels. Liver biopsies have demonstrated in such patients the presence of chronic progressive or chronic active hepatitis and cirrhosis. Severe, end-stage liver disease has been reported rarely, but the natural history of this disease in haemophilia and Christmas disease patients has not so far been clarified. Research techniques to make coagulation factor concentrates hepatitis-free are currently being investigated.
3. *Human immunodeficiency virus (HIV) infection* During the early 1980s, the majority of severely affected patients were exposed to this retrovirus which was present in factor concentrates. A particular feature of HIV infection in these patients is the rarity of Kaposi's sarcoma. Heat-treated coagulation factor concentrates have been used routinely since early 1985. It is expected that this, together with the routine screening of all blood donations, will prevent further infection in this group of patients.

Because of the above mentioned infusion-related side effects, deamino-8-D-arginine vasopressin (DDAVP), which can raise circulating factor VIII levels by its release from storage sites, should be used when possible. This is suitable treatment for mildly affected haemophiliac patients (factor VIII levels 0·1 U/ml or greater). A slow infusion of 0·3 µ/kg intravenously may allow minor surgical procedures to be performed safely. The maximum response occurs one hour after an infusion and repeated doses may be given every 6–12 hours. A diminishing response may occur after 24–48 hours, presumably due to depletion of storage sites. The side effects are water retention, mild hypotension, facial flushing and headaches. DDAVP can also be used intranasally (1–2 µg/kg). Because DDAVP activates the fibrinolytic system by the release of plasminogen activator from vascular endothelial cells, an antifibrinolytic agent, e.g. tranexamic acid, should be given simultaneously.

Patients with antibodies to factor VIII may not respond to factor concentrates. The use of porcine factor VIII, or a plasma product presumed to have factor VIII inhibitor bypassing activity (FEIBA), are frequently helpful. The activity of FEIBA is proven, but the mechanism of action remains uncertain.

Prenatal screening and antenatal testing are now available for suspected carriers of haemophilia and Christmas disease, and appropriate counselling should now be offered to all affected families.

Von Willebrand's disease (VWD)

This is probably the commonest of the hereditary coagulation disorders. The central problem for VWD patients is an abnormality, either quantitative or qualitative, of the factor VIII von Willebrand factor (VWF), a glycoprotein released from vascular endothelial cells and present in platelets and megakaryocytes. This results in a dual abnormality of platelet and coagulation function. The VWF is a large molecular weight protein which forms a dissociable complex with factor VIII coagulant protein (which is deficient in haemophiliac patients). The VWF can be measured functionally by its ability to aggregate platelets in the presence of ristocetin (ristocetin co-factor activity, RCoF) and immunologically as von Willebrand factor antigen (VWF-Ag).

VWD is a complex heterogeneous disease. The classical form (type I VWD) is usually autosomal dominant, although a severe autosomal recessive type can rarely be seen. Type I disease is due to a quantitative reduction in VWF without the presence of qualitative defects. Type II VWD includes a heterogeneous group of patients with primarily qualitative defects of VWF, although quantitative reductions in circulating protein levels are also frequently present. This group may be suspected by the presence of particularly low RCoF levels in relation to factor VIII coagulant protein and be confirmed by analysing the multimeric structure of VWF using electrophoretic techniques.

Von Willebrand's disease typically produces a mild to moderate bleeding disorder. Mucosal bleeding with epistaxis, gastrointestinal bleeding and menorrhagia is common. Bleeding may be excessive following trauma or a surgical procedure.

The diagnosis of VWD is demonstrated by:

1. A prolonged bleeding time (frequently normal in mild cases).
2. Reduced levels of factor VIII coagulant activity, VWF-Ag and RCoF activity. In vitro platelet aggregation in response to ristocetin is typically decreased.

The choice of treatment depends on the underlying severity of the disease and the clinical problem. Any treatment used should aim to correct both the prolonged bleeding time secondary to altered platelet activity and the reduced factor VIII-related activities. In practice, it is not convenient repeatedly to measure the bleeding time, and therefore one relies on factor VIII coagulant assays.

Replacement therapy may consist of the following:

1. DDAVP is effective for most cases of type I VWD. Its use in type II disease is questionable, as experience has shown that this form of treatment may not correct the bleeding time in such patients. In a particular subtype (IIB), DDAVP may actually produce aggregation of platelets in vivo with resulting thrombocytopenia.
2. For severe type I and the majority of type II patients, cryoprecipitate, which contains significant amounts of the factor VIII protein complex, is preferable in many cases, as not all factor VIII concentrates – particularly the more highly purified concentrates – are effective in these patients.

Menorrhagia may be a recurrent problem and can usually be controlled by an oestrogen preparation. Aspirin and aspirin-like drugs should be avoided, because of their inhibitory effect on platelet function. Paracetamol or codeine are suitable analgesics, having no adverse side effects on the platelet or coagulation system in moderate dosage.

ACQUIRED DISORDERS OF HAEMOSTASIS

Platelet Function Disorders

Drug-induced platelet dysfunction (Table 13.2)

Aspirin is the most important and frequently used drug in this respect. It alters platelet function by inhibiting platelet cyclo-oxygenase activity, resulting in reduced platelet prostaglandin synthesis (Fig. 13.4).

Small doses of aspirin inhibit platelet function irreversibly, and normal platelet function then depends on the production of a new cohort of platelets by megakaryocytes in the marrow, which usually takes some days. Other drugs reversibly alter platelet function and their effect diminishes once the offending agent has been withdrawn.

Platelet dysfunction associated with systemic disease (Table 13.3)

Although a mild bleeding disorder may follow, no treatment is usually necessary. Platelet transfusions are helpful, should prolonged bleeding occur. Cryoprecipitate and DDAVP have been demonstrated to be of some value in hereditary and acquired

Table 13.2
DRUGS CAUSING PLATELET DYSFUNCTION

Aspirin
Other non-steroidal anti-inflammatory drugs
Sulphinpyrazone
Alcohol
Phenothiazines
Antihistamines
Penicillin, carbenicillin
Tricyclic antidepressants

Note: These are examples, and not a complete list of drugs capable of altering platelet function.

Table 13.3
SYSTEMIC DISEASE ASSOCIATED WITH PLATELET DYSFUNCTION

Renal disease
Liver disease
Myeloproliferative diseases
Paraprotein disorders
Leukaemia and myelodysplasia

platelet dysfunctional syndromes, although their mechanism of action in this situation remains unclear.

Coagulation Disorders

Liver disease

Both quantitative and qualitative disorders of platelets and coagulation factors are present in patients with liver disease. The liver is necessary for the synthesis of coagulation factors and also for the removal of activated coagulation products from the circulation. Thrombocytopenia and platelet dysfunction may also be present. Bleeding problems are usually attributed to disordered coagulation, which may be important in increasing blood loss from bleeding oesophageal varices.

Abnormal coagulation may therefore result from:

1. Reduced synthesis of factors
2. Failure to remove activated products and FDP (which may then have an inhibitory effect on the coagulation pathway)
3. Impaired clearance of fibrinolytic enzymes, thereby increasing fibrinolysis
4. Disseminated intravascular coagulation (DIC), which frequently accompanies severe liver disease.

The vitamin K-dependent proteins, i.e. coagulation factors II (prothrombin), VII, IX and X and proteins C and S, may be reduced in patients with obstructive jaundice. Dysfibrinogenaemia, a qualitative abnormality of platelet function, occurs in the majority of patients with severe liver disease.

The prothrombin time has prognostic significance in patients with acute hepatitis and paracetamol poisoning. Marked prolongation of the prothrombin time suggests a poor prognosis for these patients

Replacement therapy is reserved for those patients with severe liver disease who are bleeding. Fresh frozen plasma ((FFP) is suitable in most situations. The corrective effect of FFP on the coagulation tests is short-lived due to the half-life of factor VII, which is only five hours. Prothrombin complex concentrates can deliver large quantities of factors II, IX and X. These should be given with caution in liver disease patients, as reports of thrombosis and DIC have occurred following their use. This may be due to the presence in the concentrate of activated coagulation factors, which would be removed from the circulation by a normal liver.

Massive transfusion syndrome

Bank blood is deficient in factors V, VIII and platelets. If a large quantity of blood is infused over a short period of time, a reduction in circulating coagulation factors and platelets will occur secondary to a dilutional effect. In severe cases, a generalized bleeding disorder occurs. Laboratory studies show a low platelet count, prolonged PT and KCCT, but the TT is normal, and this is an important point to note in distinguishing this disorder from DIC. Treatment, in the form of FFP and platelet concentrates, results in rapid correction of bleeding.

Vitamin K deficiency

Factors II, VII, IX and X and protein C and S levels may be reduced in vitamin K deficiency, which may occur in:

1. Haemorrhagic disease of the newborn
2. Malabsorption
3. Malnourished patients receiving broad spectrum antibiotics
4. Prolonged obstructive jaundice
5. Patients given vitamin K antagonists, such as warfarin
6. Patient's given certain antibiotics, e.g. cephalosporins, which may inhibit the activity of vitamin K.

Replacement treatment consists of intravenous injections of 10 mg vitamin K daily. Improvement in the coagulation parameters should occur within 6–12 hours. For immediate correction of a vitamin K-induced coagulation problem, FFP can be used.

Disseminated intravascular coagulation

DIC is a heterogeneous syndrome ranging from a subclinical disorder to severe life-threatening haemorrhage. The common pathophysiological event is the liberation into the circulation of a substance which activates the coagulation pathways. The end result is the formation of intravascular fibrin/platelet clots with secondary consumption and reduction in circulating platelets and coagulation factors. DIC is typically associated with haemorrhage, although thrombosis can occasionally be a presenting complaint. Laboratory investigation in a typical case of DIC shows:

1. Very low platelet count
2. Prolonged PT, KCCT and TT
3. Low circulating fibrinogen levels
4. Raised FDP levels.

DIC is found in the following clinical situations:

1. Infection, particularly Gram-negative bacteraemia with endotoxaemia
2. Cancer, usually associated with advanced metastatic disease or acute promyelocytic leukaemia
3. Obstetric complications, e.g. septic abortion, eclampsia, amniotic fluid embolism, abruptio placentae
4. Severe trauma or hypoxia when tissue factor is released from damaged tissues.

The treatment of DIC includes:

1. Treating the underlying cause
2. Attention to renal function and acid base balance
3. Replacement therapy with FFP, cryoprecipitate, platelet concentrates and blood transfusions
4. The use of heparin. This is controversial and there is no convincing evidence to support its use in acute DIC. Heparin may, however, be useful in those patients with chronic DIC associated with unresectable or advanced malignant disease.

Circulating anticoagulants

Acquired anticoagulants, i.e. antibodies with affinity for specific coagulation factors, occasionally occur. Those directed against factor VIII are most frequent, although antibodies directed against most of the coagulation factors have been described. Acquired factor VIII antibodies may be idiopathic or related to the use of penicillin, to rheumatoid arthritis and other collagen disorders, or to pregnancy. The clinical course is variable but frequently presents as a severe life-threatening bleeding disorder.

The lupus anticoagulant is an antibody with specificity for phospholipids and interferes with the activity of the coagulation cascade. It is frequently detected coincidentally by finding a prolonged KCCT, a normal or minimally prolonged PT, and the demonstration in the laboratory of an inhibitor with no specific activity for a particular coagulation factor. The lupus anticoagulant is perhaps a misnomer, as it occurs in many situations other than systemic lupus erythematosus. It is unusual in as much as it is not responsible for a bleeding tendency but is related to recurrent thromboses and recurrent abortions or intra-uterine death. Corticosteroids, which may suppress the activity of lupus anticoagulant, appear to be beneficial in some patients who have experienced recurrent abortions.

FURTHER READING

Hirsh J., Brain E.A. (1979). *Haemostasis and Thrombosis. A Conceptual Approach.* New York: Churchill Livingstone.

Malpass T.W., Harker L.A. (1980). Acquired disorders of platelet function. *Sem. Haematol.*, **17**, 242–256.

Thomas D., ed. (1977). Haemostasis. *Br. Med. Bull.*, **33**(3).

Voke J., Madgwick, C., Dormandy K. *Haemophilia Centre Handbook.* Immuno Ltd. Printer Flo Print, Tonbridge Wells, Kent.

Haematological Topics

Chapter Fourteen

Clinical Blood Transfusion and the Use of Blood Products

BLOOD GROUPS

Red cell blood group antigens are mainly glycoproteins and glycolipids present on the cell surface membrane and determined by autosomal genes. More than 100 blood group systems are now recognized, but only a minority are of clinical importance (Table 14.1). Antibodies to these moieties may be found in the serum of persons who lack the corresponding antigen. 'Naturally occurring' antibodies are found to the ABO antigens but are rare in most other blood group systems. 'Immune' antibodies arise by immunization of an individual by blood transfusion or by feto-maternal haemorrhage in pregnancy. Naturally occurring antibodies are usually of the IgM class (molecular weight 900 kd) and will normally agglutinate red cells in saline suspension (complete antibodies). Immune antibodies are generally of the IgG class (molecular weight 150 kd), may cross the placenta and cause fetal or neonatal haemolysis, and will not usually cause direct agglutination of red cells (incomplete antibodies). Incomplete antibodies are usually detected by the use of antiglobulin reagents (indirect antiglobulin or Coombs' test) or using specifically treated red cells (enzyme-treated or in albumin suspension).

ABO BLOOD GROUP SYSTEM

Groups A, B, AB and O are determined by the presence of the relevant antigens on the red cell surface. Except in neonates,

Table 14.1
SOME MAJOR BLOOD GROUP SYSTEMS

Name	Antigen
ABO	A B (H-sustance)
Rhesus	C c D E e
Kell	K k
Lewis	Le^a Le^b
P	P_1 P P^k
I	I i
Lutheran	Lu^a Lu^b
Duffy	Fy^a Fy^b
Kidd	JK^a JK^b
MNSs	M N S s

naturally occurring antibodies to the appropriate ABO antigens are found in the serum (Table 14.2). This system is of clinical importance, as a major ABO mismatch transfusion (A into O or B; B into O or A; AB into O, A or B) can produce a serious haemolytic transfusion reaction with destruction of the transfused cells. As antibodies present in transfused blood are rapidly diluted, it was common to regard patients of group O as 'universal donors' and group AB as 'universal recipients'. This is potentially dangerous as a proportion of donors (particularly of group O) possess 'immune' IgG anti-A or -B or high titre naturally occurring antibodies sufficient to cause significant haemolysis of recipient red cells. Modern rapid cross-matching techniques, and increased use of the policy of 'grouping and

Table 14.2
ABO BLOOD GROUP SYSTEM

Blood group	Red cell antigens	Serum antibodies	Frequency in UK population
O	NIL	anti-A + anti-B	47%
A	A	anti-B	42%
B	B	anti-A	8%
AB	A + B	NIL	3%

antibody screening' surgical and obstetric patients before admission, make it possible to give blood of the same ABO group in most emergency situations.

RHESUS (Rh) BLOOD GROUP SYSTEM

This is a rather poorly understood blood group system determined by three alternative genes (alleles), C/c, D/d and E/e, of which D produces the most powerful antigen and is of major clinical importance (d antigen probably does not exist). About 85 per cent of the indigenous British population possess the D antigen (Rh(D) positive), although there is wide geographic variation throughout the world. Antirhesus antibodies in the serum nearly always arise after immunization by transfusion or pregnancy. Transfusion of D-positive red cells into a person with immune anti-D antibodies can cause a severe haemolytic reaction and all blood donations are routinely Rh-typed ('rhesus negative' donor blood is cde/cde). IgG anti-D may cross the placenta and was formerly a major cause of haemolytic disease of the newborn.

WHITE CELL ANTIGENS

ABO and certain other 'red cell' antigens are also found on leucocytes, but the most clinically important white cell antigens belong to the human leucocyte-A (HLA) system. The HLA-A, B, C and Dr antigens, determined by genes on chromosome 6, are an integral part of the process of cell-cell interaction and antigen-processing by the cellular immune system. HLA antigens are present on most nucleated cells, and HLA-incompatibility is a major barrier to certain types of organ transplantation. HLA antibodies arise by immunization after transfusion or pregnancy and are an important cause of febrile transfusion reactions.

PLATELET ANTIGENS

In addition to ABO and HLA antigens, certain 'platelet-specific' antigens are known. Of most clinical significance is the Pl^{A1} antigen which is present in more than 95 per cent of the British population. The rare Pl^{A1} negative mother, immunized by prior transfusion or pregnancy, can transmit IgG anti-Pl^{A1} across the placenta and cause iso-immune neonatal thrombocytopenia.

BLOOD PRODUCTS FOR TRANSFUSION

'Whole blood' collected into an anticoagulant solution at blood donor sessions is now increasingly being divided into a variety of components at the Blood Transfusion Centre and at central plasma fractionation laboratories. This process, facilitated by modern plastic collection packs, allows the harvesting of labile plasma and cellular components which would otherwise be wasted during storage. The demand for plasma components, such as factor VIII for the treatment of haemophilia, is in excess of red cell requirements and many centres now collect plasma alone from certain donors using automated 'cell-separators'. The efficient economy of blood usage requires intelligent selection of appropriate blood products by the clinician and avoidance of the wasteful use of 'whole blood'.

Red Cells

'Whole blood' consists of about 420 ml of donor blood and 120 ml of anticoagulant solution. Traditional acid citrate dextrose (ACD) anticoagulant is now rapidly being superseded by citrate phosphate dextrose plus adenine (CPD-A), which allows a longer shelf-life at 4 °C (35–42 days). CPD-A better maintains the level of 2,3-diphosphoglycerate and improves the metabolic function of stored red cells. The activity of granulocytes, platelets and labile coagulation factors is very low after a few days of storage. The main clinical indication for the transfusion of whole blood is replacement of acute surgical or obstetric haemorrhage.

'Concentrated red cells' (synonym, packed red cells) are produced by removing variable amounts of plasma from whole blood. Chronically anaemic patients have a normal or expanded plasma volume, and transfusion of concentrated red cells produces less risk of circulatory overload. The plasma removed from red cell concentrates may be replaced by a mixture of saline, adenine, glucose and mannitol (SAG-M), which results in a less viscous product for transfusion and good preservation of red cell metabolism. The removed plasma is used for fractionation.

White cell-depleted blood is used to prevent febrile reactions and to reduce the rate of HLA sensitization in patients who are candidates for organ transplantation or who require long-term transfusion support (e.g. thalassaemia major or aplastic anaemia). Methods available for white cell depletion, in ascending order of efficiency and expense, include in-line micro-aggregate filters at the bedside, cotton wool filtration in the laboratory, and the use of frozen, reconstituted red cells. Patients may become refractory to random platelet donations because of the development of HLA antibodies. Efficient and convenient methods of white cell depletion of platelet concentrates by filtration or centrifugation are increasingly available and may be used to abrogate febrile reactions and reduce the risk of allo-immunization.

Platelet Concentrates

These are usually obtained from individual blood donations by centrifugation of plasma. The therapeutic dose of platelets for an adult is usually 4–6 pooled donors units per day. Only platelets of groups O and A are routinely collected, and cross-matching is not required. Stored platelets are viable for 3–7 days at room temperature, depending on the type of collection pack and anticoagulant used. Single donor platelets, obtained by apheresis on a cell-separator, are now increasingly available. Platelets may be given therapeutically, in response to bleeding in a thrombocytopenic patient, or prophylactically (commonly when the platelet count falls below $20 \times 10^9/1$).

Plasma Components

Whole fresh frozen plasma (FFP) may be used as a source of all coagulation factors, but the volumes required make it an inferior product for the treatment of specific factor deficiencies. Much of the fresh plasma collected is frozen and sent to fractionation laboratories for the manufacture of a range of products (Table 14.3). The greatest demand is for factor VIII used in the treatment of haemophilia-A.

Table 14.3
PRODUCTS OF PLASMA FRACTIONATION

Product	Contents	Possible clinical use
Fresh frozen plasma (FFP)	All coagulation factors	Liver disease DIC Massive transfusion Warfarin overdose
Cryoprecipitate	Factor VIII Fibrinogen	Haemophilia-A Von Willebrand's disease DIC
Factor VIII concentrate	Factor VIII	Haemophilia-A
Factor IX concentrate	Factor IX	Haemophilia-B (Christmas disease)
Factors II, VII, IX, X concentrate	Most products contain mainly II, IX and X	Liver disease* Warfarin overdose Acquired factor II, IX or X deficiency
Antithrombin III concentrate	ATIII	ATIII deficiency DIC
Human albumin solutions	5% or 20% ('salt poor') solutions	Plasma expansion/replacement Hypoalbuminaemia in liver or renal disease No risk of hepatitis or AIDS
Immunoglobulin fractions:– (Older products were for intramuscular injection only. New intravenous products now available)	'Normal' immunoglobulin 'Hyperimmune' immunoglobulin	Immunodeficiency syndromes Hepatitis-A Hepatitis-B Varicella-zoster Measles Cytomegalovirus Rabies etc.

Product	Contents	Possible clinical use
	Anti-Rh (D)	Prophylaxis of haemolytic disease of the newborn
	Intravenous immunoglobulin (IVIG)	Immunodeficiency Idiopathic thrombocytopenic purpura

*Some of these products carry high risk of thrombosis. AIDS = acquired immunodeficiency syndrome; DIC = disseminated intravascular coagulation; Rh = rhesus.

COMPLICATIONS OF BLOOD TRANSFUSION AND THEIR PREVENTION

Haemolytic Transfusion Reactions

These are usually due to the transfusion of blood incompatible for the ABO or Rh groups. Serious reactions usually result from the destruction of donor red cells by antibodies in the recipient's plasma. Clerical or administrative errors in the laboratory or ward are probably the most common cause of incompatible transfusion, and careful and rigorous checking procedures are necessary at all stages. There is a wide variation in the clinical severity of haemolytic transfusion reactions, from those which are fatal to the clinically inapparent. Early symptoms and signs may include pain or heat along the vein, lumbar pain, headache, fever, hypotension and chills. Serious reactions may include the development of shock and disseminated intravascular coagulation (DIC), with haemorrhage from surgical wounds and acute renal failure due to tubular necrosis. The early features may easily be missed in patients under general anaesthesia. The extent of haemolysis may be indicated by the presence of haemoglobinuria (often transient) and jaundice. At its most mild, the destruction of even a large amount of incompatible blood may only be evidenced by a failure in the predicted rise in post-transfusion haemoglobin level and the development of jaundice on the day after transfusion. Delayed transfusion reactions are usually clinically mild and are due to a secondary immune response occurring in a patient sensitized by previous transfusion.

They result in a fall in haemoglobin or jaundice occurring up to two weeks after transfusion.

The laboratory diagnosis of a haemolytic transfusion reaction includes rechecking the patient and donor groups and cross-match (using the pretransfusion patient sample), and seeking evidence of intravascular haemolysis (haemoglobinuria, haemoglobinaemia, raised bilirubin, reduced haptoglobins) and DIC.

Treatment includes the immediate cessation of transfusion, maintenance of blood pressure with plasma volume expanders, treatment of clinically apparent DIC with appropriate replacement therapy, and standard medical treatment for acute renal failure.

Allergic Reactions

Allergic reactions during transfusion are common and often due to antigens on transfused donor leucocytes (commonly HLA antigens) or plasma proteins. Reactions vary from fever and chills to severe angio-oedema and anaphylaxis. The transfusion of white cell-depleted blood (see above) will usually ameliorate or prevent such reactions and the use of 20 micron micro-aggregate filters with FFP has been highly effective, presumably by removing white cell debris.

Transmission of Infection

The transmission of infection by blood transfusion is assuming increasing importance. Bacterial contamination is very rare in blood which has been correctly collected and stored but may be rapidly fatal if the unit is transfused. Among the viruses which may be transmitted by blood products, are hepatitis-B, hepatitis non-A, non-B, human immunodeficiency virus (HIV) and cytomegalovirus (CMV). Donors in developed countries are now routinely screened for hepatitis-B_S antigen and for antibodies to HIV. Products such as factor VIII concentrate derived from large donor pools (often several thousand donors) are a particular risk, although recent developments in 'heat treatment' may significantly reduce the risk of viral transmission. Albumin solutions, Purified Protein Fraction (PPF) and intravenous immunoglobulin solutions seem to be largely free of risk. Current concerns include the late sequelae of transfusion-acquired non-A non-B hepatitis (cirrhosis, hepatocellular carcinoma) and the inability of present techniques to detect variant HIV species. CMV transmission is a particular risk to immunosuppressed transplant recipients, and many centres are now establishing pools of donors serologically negative for CMV antibodies. CMV is transmitted by contaminating white cells, and filtered blood products may be protective. Other infections potentially transmissible by transfusion include syphilis (all donors routinely screened), malaria, brucellosis and infectious mononucleosis.

Circulatory Overload

Circulatory overload causing acute pulmonary oedema is a particular risk in the elderly, in neonates and in patients with severe megaloblastic anaemia, and is probably the commonest cause of death following transfusion. Stringent criteria for transfusion, the use of concentrated red cells, careful monitoring and the use of diuretics or partial red cell exchange transfusion (manual or on an automated cell-separator), where appropriate, will reduce the incidence of this complication.

Air Embolism

This is much less common since plastic transfusion packs replaced glass bottles with air inlets. Accidental disconnection of central venous catheters may now be the commonest cause. Clinical symptoms of significant air embolism include cyanosis, dyspnoea and syncope. Immediate treatment measures include placing the patient head down on the left side to deviate intracardiac air bubbles away from the right ventricular outflow tract.

'Massive Transfusion'

Massive transfusion, equivalent to the circulating blood volume or more, may produce a variety of problems. The rapid transfusion of stored blood may produce a fall in plasma ionized calcium levels due to the citrate anticoagulant. As stored blood ages, potassium is released from red cells into the plasma, and significant hyperkalaemia may occur from rapid, massive transfusion. These problems are exacerbated by coexisting hepatic or renal dysfunction, and cardiac arrhythmias or arrest may occur. Such massive transfusions may also impair haemostasis by the dilution of platelets and coagulation factors. Measures to reduce these problems include the prophylactic administration of FFP and platelet concentrates and the use of relatively fresh or metabolically active red cells (red cells stored in CPD-A anticoagulant are significantly better in this respect). Ultra-fresh blood, less than 24 hours old, is now rarely available, in view of the necessity for HIV and hepatitis testing, and carries a significantly higher risk of transmitting CMV infection.

Iron Overload

This is a complication of long-term transfusion support, largely seen in patients with β-thalassaemia major, aplastic anaemia or sideroblastic anaemia. There are no specific excretory mechanisms for iron, and life-threatening clinical problems result from its deposition in the myocardium, liver and endocrine organs, such as the pancreas. The mechanism of organ damage by iron is probably the peroxidation of lipid in biological membranes. Chelation therapy with daily subcutaneous infusion of desferrioxamine should be considered in all such patients and produces significant prolongation of life in patients with thalassaemia major.

Post-Transfusion Purpura

This is a rare cause of severe thrombocytopenia developing within 7–10 days of blood transfusion. Such patients have usually been multiparous women, and serological investigations demonstrate the presence of anti-platelet antibodies, usually anti-Pl^{A1}. The patient's own platelets are usually negative for this antigen, and it is assumed that they were sensitized by previous pregnancy or blood transfusion and that the rise in antibody is due to a secondary immune response. Why this antibody should cause autologous platelet destruction is not clear, but the severity of thrombocytopenia may be clinically hazardous and persist for several weeks. Treatment measures include exchange transfusion or the administration of high-dose intravenous immunoglobulin.

FURTHER READING

Mollison P.L., Engelfreit C.P., Contreras M. (1987). *Blood Transfusion in Clinical Medicine*, 8th edn. Oxford and Edinburgh: Blackwell Scientific Publications.

Worlledge S. (1981). Practical blood transfusions. In *Postgraduate Haematology* (Hoffbrand A.V., Lewis S.M., eds.). London: Heinemann Medical Books, pp. 347–379.

Chapter Fifteen

Acute Leukaemia

DEFINITION

Acute leukaemia is an uncontrolled clonal proliferation of haemopoietic stem cells, resulting in replacement of the normal marrow cells and infiltration of organs by stem cells. In the pretreatment era, acute leukaemias were distinguished from chronic leukaemias by their short history of onset (a few weeks, compared with many months) and rapid death (within three months, compared with chronic leukaemias where patients may live for some years without treatment).

BACKGROUND

Aetiology

In most cases of acute leukaemia, there is no obvious cause and no family history. Irradiation after nuclear explosions and for treatment of ankylosing spondylitis have been associated with an increased incidence of acute myeloid leukaemia a few years later. Previous chemotherapy, particularly if associated with radiotherapy, undoubtedly predisposes to acute leukaemia, e.g. in Hodgkin's disease, polycythaemia rubra vera and myeloma. Viral infection has been implicated in some animal leukaemias, and HTLV-1, a retrovirus, has been isolated from a particular form of T-cell acute lymphoblastic leukaemia found in Japan and the West Indies. Modern cytogenetic studies reveal non-random chromosomal abnormalities in the majority of patients with acute leukaemia, and some of these are associated with rearrangements of oncogenes. Congenital disorders such as Down's syndrome, and rare disorders like Fanconi's anaemia, Wiskott–Aldrich and

Bloom's syndrome, show a clear increase in the incidence of acute leukaemia.

Incidence

Acute lymphoblastic leukaemia (ALL) is a rare disease with perhaps 300 new cases diagnosed yearly in the UK, but the incidence of the disease peaks in children where it is the commonest cause of malignancy.

In adults, acute myeloid leukaemia (AML) is about five times as common as acute lymphoblastic leukaemia, and there is a great increase in incidence with increasing age, particularly over 50 years old. The incidence is rising but is currently about three new cases per year per 100 000 population in the West, where it accounts for about three per cent of all malignancies in adults.

PATHOLOGY

Instead of the marrow stem cells dividing and differentiating into a variety of mature red cells, white cells and platelets, the stem cells themselves proliferate in acute leukaemia, replacing the marrow and often spilling into the blood as blast cells. The name 'leukaemia' reflects this increase in the white cells in the blood. Only when the number of blasts in the body has reached about 10^{12} do patients become ill with anaemia, bleeding and susceptibility to infection. With treatment, reduction of the leukaemic mass to about 10^{10} restores health to normal, and conventional marrow examination appears normal at this point.

SYMPTOMS AND SIGNS

Acute leukaemia usually presents with a history of a few weeks of non-specific illness, loss of appetite and symptoms of anaemia. There may be no other symptoms or signs to suggest leukaemia, or there may be problems associated with bleeding, infection or, less commonly, infiltration.

Thrombocytopenia may cause skin and mucosal bleeding, with purpura, bruising, epistaxis, bleeding gums, gastro-intestinal haemorrhage, haematuria and sometimes haemoptysis. Occasionally, cerebral haemorrhage occurs, and the fundi should always be examined for signs of haemorrhage.

Neutropenia renders patients susceptible to pyogenic infections, particularly of the lungs, mucous membranes and skin. Fever usually reflects infection, but the classical signs of inflammation, such as erythema, tenderness, swelling and production of pus (or purulent sputum), may be minimal because of the neutropenia. Untreated local sepsis can rapidly extend to a fatal septicaemia. The mouth and throat should be examined with care for signs of ulceration, candida and herpes. The perineum should be observed for signs of infection, but rectal examination is generally avoided, as this can actually provoke serious perineal infection or even septicaemia.

Lymphadenopathy and hepatosplenomegaly from leukaemic infiltration is generally less pronounced than with the chronic leukaemias, but may be impressive in T-cell ALL, with young patients presenting with mediastinal obstruction by lymph nodes. Infiltration of bones and joints may cause pain, particularly in children, but testicular involvement is usually painless. Gum hypertrophy is classically found in acute monocytic leukaemia and infiltration of the skin may cause painless, raised, violaceous lesions.

INVESTIGATIONS

The diagnosis is usually made by examination of the blood and confirmed by marrow examination.

Anaemia may be severe and is usually normocytic. It reflects failure of marrow production and is compounded by bleeding. The platelet count is greatly reduced in most patients, but the leucocyte count is variable. If the marrow is releasing large numbers of leukaemic cells, the total white count is greatly increased and consists mostly of blasts, but usually the absolute neutrophil count is reduced. The risk of pyogenic infection reflects the severity of the neutropenia. Serious infection is unusual with neutrophil counts above $0.5 \times 10^9/1$, but is frequent as the count falls below $0.2 \times 10^9/1$. In a few patients, the marrow does not release the blast cells into the blood (giving rise to the ugly term 'aleukaemic leukaemia'), and in this case the white cell count will be below normal, reflecting the low numbers of neutrophils. In such cases, the diagnosis can be made only by marrow examination, which is abnormal in acute leukaemia with replacement of the normal range of marrow cells by sheets of blast cells.

The type of acute leukaemia is initially determined by the appearance of blast cells in a Romanovsky stained blood or marrow film, aided by special stains, e.g. myeloperoxidase which shows positive cytoplasmic granules only in AML. Separation of ALL and AML is of great importance, as the appropriate treatment is very different. The Romanovsky stain is available worldwide and is the basis of the French/American/British (FAB) cooperative group classification (see Table 15.1), which separates ALL into subtypes L1, L2 and L3, and AML into subtypes M1 to M6. This classification of ALL is of limited use, and a subclassification based on monoclonal marker studies of the surface, nucleus and cytoplasm of the blast cells is shown in Table 15.2. Detailed chromosomal analysis may be helpful, as recognition of subtypes of the broad divisions may be important for guiding the details of treatment strategies. For example, cases with the t(15:17) translocation, previously often diagnosed as M5, are now recognized as a hypogranular variation of M3 and should probably be treated

Table 15.1
FAB CLASSIFICATION OF ACUTE LEUKAEMIA
(based on Romanovsky stained film)

Acute lymphoblastic leukaemia (ALL)
L1 Lymphoblasts with scant (<20%) cytoplasm and regular nuclei
L2 Lymphoblasts of variable size, >20% cytoplasm and often a cleft nucleus
L3 Large lymphoblasts, cytoplasm basophilic with vacuolation

Acute myeloid leukaemia (AML)
M1 Myeloblastic without maturation (but >3% myeloid markers)
M2 Granulocytic with some maturation (50% blasts and promyelocytes)
M3 Hypergranular with multiple Auer rods
M4 Myelomonocytic (with >20% monocytes and >20% early myeloid cells)
M5 Monocytic (with most cells monocytic, <20% myeloid markers)
M6 Erythroleukaemia (>10% pro-erythroblasts, and erythroid dysplasia)

FAB = French/American/British.

Table 15.2
CLASSIFICATION OF ALL
(based on cell marker studies)

Leukaemia	Nuclear TdT	_____ Cell surface CD _____								Cytoplasmic CD		
		10	34	19	DR	7	22	13	33	3	22	IgM
ALL type												
cALL	+	+	+	(+)	(+)	−	−	−	−	−	+	−
Null ALL	+	−	−	+	+	−	−	−	−	−	(+)	−
T-ALL	+	−	−	−	−	+	−	−	−	+	−	−
Pre-B	+	−	−	+	(+)	−	−	−	−	−	(+)	+
B-cell	−	−	−	+	(+)	−	+	−	−	−	−	−
AML	−	−	−	−	(+)	−	−	+	+	−	−	−

ALL = acute lymphoblastic leukaemia; AML = acute myeloid leukaemia; cALL = common ALL; CD = cluster designation; TdT = terminal deoxynucleotidyl transferase.

The table shows the immunophenotypes of ALL demonstrated by monoclonal antibodies. These recognize antigen determinants (on the surface, nucleus and cytoplasm of lymphoid cells), which reflect maturity and differentiation. The numbers refer to the agreed cluster designation (CD numbers). IgM refers to μ heavy chains. Results of less importance in diagnosis are shown in parentheses.

In general, the cytoplasmic studies are more difficult but extremely sensitive and can detect as few as 1/1000 cells. The subtypes normally exhibit at least two distinctive antigens, which enables characterization even if the expression of one antigen is poor.

In most cases of ALL, the cells lack B- or T-cell differentiation, but express an antigen initially known as common ALL antigen (CALLA) and recognized by an antibody raised in rabbits. CD10 is a monoclonal antibody which recognizes a similar antigen. Common ALL (cALL) accounts for about 70 per cent, T-cell 10 per cent, and B-cell five per cent of cases of ALL.

A number of acute leukaemias are now being recognized which show a mixed appearance with combinations of more than one type of acute leukaemia.

with heparin to control the problem of disseminated intravascular coagulation (DIC) associated with M3 leukaemias.

It is usual to measure blood urea, potassium and other electrolytes, uric acid, and liver function, which may be deranged before or during treatment. Abnormalities in coagulation may be found if there is liver damage (e.g. from drugs or septicaemia), and this may exacerbate bleeding from thrombocytopenia. Evidence of DIC should be sought in patients with promyelocytic leukaemia (M3). The problem can lead to severe haemorrhage during the first few days of treatment, when the cell breakdown releases thrombogenic factors.

The investigation of infective problems follows standard lines, but should be pursued with speed and care in view of the fact that infection can be rapidly fatal in these patients. As treatment should not be delayed in patients with pyrexia, it is usual to take blood, urine and swabs from other possible sites of infection for culture, and then to start treatment with intravenous broad spectrum antibiotics (chosen with knowledge of local hospital pathogens) before any results become available. Treatment may then be modified later in the light of culture and sensitivity results.

DIFFERENTIAL DIAGNOSIS

The presentation symptoms are often non-specific and may initially mimic virus infections and other diseases. Once blood is examined, the diagnosis is usually obvious. In the uncommon patients with pancytopenia and no blasts in the blood (*see* Chapter 9 for other causes of pancytopenia), marrow examination is needed to reveal the diagnosis. On occasions, the diagnosis of the type and subtype of acute leukaemia present may give the haematologist considerable difficulty.

TREATMENT

In 1948, aminopterin – a folic acid antagonist – was shown temporarily to improve the condition of children with ALL. Since then, the results of treatment of leukaemia have steadily improved. These improvements have followed the introduction of new chemotherapeutic drugs (and their detailed scheduling and assessment by specialist centres) and great improvements in supportive care, particularly in relation to good nursing, antibiotic regimens and blood product support in patients rendered severely pancytopenic and immunosuppressed by chemotherapy.

Where possible, patients with acute leukaemia should be referred to specialist centres, where the aim of treatment is cure. Patients are generally better able to cope with the very demanding treatment if the diagnosis, aims, outline and expected complications of treatment are discussed with them and their families.

The drugs used now in treating acute leukaemia cause vomiting, temporary hair loss and reduced fertility. The marrow is usually rendered temporarily aplastic. Anaemia is treated by red cell transfusions, and bleeding problems from thrombocytopenia are usually controlled by daily platelet transfusions. Neutropenia increases the risk and severity of bacterial infection (*see* above). Methods to prevent infection, and rapid and appropriate treatment of any infections that develop, have made a great impact on survival. Some degree of temporary organ damage (especially lung, kidney, liver, heart, gastro-intestinal tract and brain) and electrolyte disturbance is common with the intensive regimens now used.

Acute Lymphoblastic Leukaemia

Suitable drugs for treating ALL became available first, and traditional treatment could be separated into four phases: remission induction, consolidation, central nervous system (CNS) prophylaxis, and maintenance. Late intensification is a more recent concept.

Remission

Remission is usually defined by the return of the blood counts to normal and a marrow showing blast cell numbers under five per cent, and this stage is essential if patients are to do well long-term. The use of oral prednisolone and weekly intravenous vincristine was found to induce a remission within four weeks in most children with ALL. The therapeutic ratio is high with very little damage to the normal stem cells, so that after a few days, the child can normally be treated on an out-patient basis. The patient enters remission, and his health usually returns to normal when the number of leukaemic cells has been reduced from about 10^{12} at presentation to 10^{10}.

Consolidation

If treatment is stopped at this point, the leukaemic cells rapidly return and the patient relapses. Further courses of treatment with drugs similar to those used for induction are given as consolidation to reduce the leukaemic cell mass further in order to prevent early relapse.

CNS prophylaxis

With prolongation of life by such remission induction and consolidation treatment, a new complication arose in over half the children with ALL, namely CNS relapse, presenting with headaches, neck stiffness, fits and various neurological problems. The blood–brain barrier prevents most chemotherapeutic drugs from reaching the CNS, and so the leukaemic cells usually seen in small numbers at presentation are able to proliferate undisturbed. The incidence of this complication can be reduced to about five per cent by irradiation of the brain (with 18–24 Gy) and a series of intrathecal methotrexate injections. During the radiation, children may be nauseated and drowsy, and after a few weeks, complete alopecia develops. The hair later regrows completely normally, but wigs, hats and scarves can be useful temporarily. The radiation somnolence syndrome is seen in most patients and occurs three to seven weeks after treatment, causing drowsiness, nausea and irritability lasting one to two weeks. Leucoencephalopathy causes a variety of serious CNS complications, but is usually seen only after larger than normal doses of methotrexate or radiotherapy, or where recurrent CNS leukaemia has developed.

Maintenance

Maintenance therapy was designed to eliminate completely 'minimal residual disease', a term applied to the few residual leukaemic cells which sometimes persist after initial treatment and which may be responsible for subsequent relapse. Drugs shown to be active at this stage, such as oral 6-mercaptopurine and methotrexate, are given over a period of 18 to 24 months on a regular out-patient basis.

Modern approaches to chemotherapy in ALL

Many specialist centres are now using very intensive but short induction treatment schedules in the hope of achieving a greater leukaemic cell kill at the cost of prolonged periods of drug-induced aplasia. Drugs such as asparaginase, daunorubicin, VP-

16 and doxorubicin (Adriamycin) have been added early in treatment to vincristine and steroids, and with this intensive treatment, patients are more nauseated and made severely pancytopenic, requiring hospitalization for some weeks. Remission rates of over 95 per cent are achieved in children, but in adults the rate is nearer 75 per cent. CNS prophylaxis may be followed by further intensive treatment, now referred to as 'intensification' (early, late or both). The value of maintenance treatment with these intensive schedules is unknown.

Early deaths from septicaemia and organ toxicity remain a problem. Later deaths from pneumocystis pneumonitis are preventable by cotrimoxazole prophylaxis, and the unacceptably high death rate from measles infection in the UK would be entirely preventable by a high uptake of vaccination in the community. Despite these difficulties, early results encourage the belief that the overall cure rate, even in poor-risk patients (males over 15 years old with a leucocyte count above $20 \times 10^9/l$ at presentation), will be improved. The appealing concept that good-risk patients (e.g. girls under 15 years old with a leucocyte count under $10 \times 10^9/l$ at presentation) can be adequately treated by more gentle chemotherapy, which would reduce iatrogenic deaths, does not appear to be valid.

Acute Myeloid Leukaemia

Unfortunately, with AML the therapeutic ratio is very low, and if drugs are used in sufficient doses to eradicate the leukaemic cells (as required for cure), the normal stem cells are completely destroyed and the patient dies from aplasia. Large, but just sublethal, doses of combinations of drugs are given over a few days in hospital, separated by short intervals during which the normal stem cells recover faster than the leukaemic cells. With the next course of treatment, the leukaemic cells start at only a fraction of their initial level and become reduced even further. About 65 per cent of adults (more if young, less if old) go into remission after one to three courses of intensive combinations of drugs such as daunorubicin, cytosine arabinoside and 6-thioguanine (DAT).

Consolidation treatment is given after remission has been achieved with, perhaps, two courses of different combinations of drugs (e.g. chosen from VP-16, cyclophosphamide, M-AMSA, mitozantrone and steroids), and this again usually requires some weeks of in-patient treatment.

CNS leukaemia is relatively uncommon in AML (but does occur with some varieties, such as monocytic leukaemia), and maintenance therapy appears to offer no survival advantage (but is toxic and unpleasant to receive). Late intensification may have some long-term value in AML, but is still being assessed. Our thoughts on chemotherapy schedules are likely to be changed by the introduction of transplantation (*see* below).

COMPLICATIONS

If patients do not go into remission with initial chemotherapy, they die rapidly from bleeding or infection. Some patients whose leukaemia is responding to chemotherapy may die from infection or from the toxic effects of the intense initial treatment.

The major problem with patients who enter remission and return to normal life is the likelihood of the disease recurring after some months or years, usually in the marrow. In ALL, there is also a tendency for the disease to relapse in the CNS and, in males, in the testes.

TRANSPLANTATION

The concept of transplantation is simple. The high doses of chemotherapy and radiotherapy required to eliminate the leukaemic cell line completely are given in the knowledge that this would cause fatal aplasia by destroying the normal stem cells. The patient is then rescued from this lethal aplasia by the introduction of healthy compatible marrow cells. About 3×10^8 nucleated cells per kilogram of recipient (usually 500 to 1000 ml of marrow in adults) are aspirated from the donor's posterior iliac crests and then transfused into the recipient by vein. The stem cells find their way to the marrow, and after a few weeks, marrow function starts to return.

Bone marrow transplantation may be allogeneic (from a HLA-matched sibling or even a HLA-matched but unrelated donor), autologous (from the patient himself after he has entered complete remission), or syngeneic (if there is an identical twin). With syngeneic and autologous transplants, the immediate mortality is fairly low, but the major complication is of later relapse of the leukaemia. With allogeneic transplantation, there is a significant problem with graft-*versus*-host disease (*see* below), but the risk of leukaemic relapse is lower.

Allogeneic Transplantation

Compatible sibling transplantation (from an HLA-matched donor)

Allogeneic bone marrow transplantation is now an established treatment for patients under 50 years old with acute leukaemia and with chronic granulocytic leukaemia in the chronic phase. Whilst it is currently the treatment of choice for AML, it is not generally considered appropriate for patients under 15 years of age with ALL, as better results are obtained with modern chemotherapy schedules. It is therefore used for patients with ALL who are known to fare badly with conventional treatment, e.g. patients over 15 (but under 50) years of age or those with relapsed disease. The indications for transplantation in leukaemia have changed in the last few years and will doubtless continue to change with advances in both conventional and transplantation techniques.

Patients undergoing a transplant usually require about six weeks in hospital with intensive support. The dangers of the procedure are considerable and include toxic effects of the drugs and radiotherapy on the lungs and other organs, profound neutropenia during the first few weeks (with its risks of pyogenic infections), immunosuppression for about six months after a transplant (rendering the patient vulnerable to all types of infection, including opportunistic infections such as cytomegalovirus and fungal infections), and graft-*versus*-host disease (*see* below). Recurrence of the leukaemia is clearly less likely than with conventional treatment.

Graft-*versus*-host disease (GVHD) occurs to a minor extent in most patients and reflects the recognition by the new marrow that it is surrounded by a 'foreign' body, which it attempts to destroy. It is mediated by T-lymphocytes of donor origin. The acute form of GVHD presents with fever and an erythematous itchy rash on the palms, soles and elsewhere, and sometimes with jaundice, diarrhoea, nausea and abdominal pain. The chronic form of

GVHD presents later with a variety of systemic problems, which may include dryness and thickening of the skin, lichen planus, arthritis, contractures, malabsorption, liver failure and lung problems. Mild degrees of GVHD are associated with a low incidence of recurrence of leukaemia, but more severe forms can be fatal. Attempts to prevent GVHD by T-cell depletion of the marrow donation have had some success, but this has been marred by problems with failure of engraftment.

HLA-matched unrelated donor transplants and mismatched transplantation

A severe limitation to allogeneic transplantation is that only patients under about 50 years old can be treated and that only one in four siblings is fully compatible as donor. Results using very minor incompatibilities (e.g. haplo-identical with one mismatch) are now good and increase the theoretical chances of finding a donor to about 47 per cent, but the results of greater mismatches continue to be unacceptable.

An interesting and possibly important development is the use of HLA-matched unrelated donors (MUD) from a panel. Results with this technique are currently not as good as those using HLA-matched siblings, but they look interesting for certain diseases, such as chronic granulocytic leukaemia, where autologous transplantation is not helpful. A pool of 250 000 donors, which is quite feasible in the UK, is needed to find fully HLA-matched donors for about 60 per cent of patients, and this number would increase significantly if minor incompatibilities prove acceptable.

Autologous transplantation

The role of autologous transplantation in patients who have no HLA-matched sibling donor is now being assessed in the treatment of AML (under 55 years old) and ALL (15–55 years old), and early results are encouraging.

Marrow is harvested from patients who have entered remission and is stored temporarily while the patient is given high-dose chemotherapy and/or radiotherapy to eradicate as far as possible any leukaemic cells remaining in the body. The patient is then rescued from the resulting aplasia by infusion of the stored marrow (which in remission should be virtually free of leukaemic cells).

Compared with allogeneic transplantation, there is virtually no GVHD, and there is less immune suppression and infection. Unfortunately, a greater relapse rate is seen later, but this is likely to prove less than with conventional chemotherapy.

PROGNOSIS

Untreated patients with acute leukaemia usually die within three months of presentation. In children with ALL, modern treatment schedules are curing over 50 per cent of patients. ALL in adults is more difficult to treat than in children, and adult AML is yet more challenging. Some groups are now recording 25 per cent five-year survival with standard chemotherapy, but it is still not certain that these patients will not relapse later, as earlier trials show continuing relapses even 10 years after initial remission, so that survival falls to about 10 per cent at 10 years. With allogeneic transplantation, the cure rate is about 50 per cent. The long-term survival with autotransplantation is being assessed, with good initial results.

With modern treatment, the difference in survival between different subtypes of leukaemia is not as pronounced as previously, but the prognosis with B-cell ALL and with the blastic crisis of chronic granulocytic leukaemia (*see* Chapter 16) remains extremely poor.

FURTHER READING

Bennett J.M., Catovsky D., Daniel M-T., et al. (1976). Proposals for the classification of the acute leukaemias. *Br. J. Haemat.*, **33**, 451–458.

Blume K.G., Petz L.D., eds. (1983). *Clinical Bone Marrow Transplantation.* New York: Churchill Livingstone.

Chessels J.M. (1985). Risks and benefits of intensive treatment of acute leukaemia. *Arch. Dis. Child.*, **60**, 193–195.

Goldman J.M., Preisler H.D., eds. (1984). *Leukaemias.* London: Butterworths.

Chapter Sixteen

The Chronic Leukaemias

In the pretreatment era, chronic leukaemias were distinguished from the 'acute' leukaemias by their more indolent course and prolonged survival.

CHRONIC MYELOID LEUKAEMIA

Definition

Chronic myeloid leukaemia (CML; synonym, chronic granulocytic leukaemia) is a malignant haematological disorder characterized by a relatively indolent 'chronic phase' with proliferation of both mature and immature cells of the myeloid series followed by transformation to an acute leukaemia ('acute phase').

Background

The aetiology of CML is unknown, although an increased incidence was seen in survivors of the atomic bomb explosions in Japan. The incidence is about one in 100 000 persons per year, comprising 20–30 per cent of all cases of leukaemia. Median age of onset is the mid-forties, and the sex incidence is equal.

Pathology

Several lines of evidence show that at the time of presentation virtually all haemopoietic cells belong to the malignant clone. That the malignant transformation occurs at the level of a primitive pluripotential cell is confirmed by transformation to acute lymphoblastic leukaemia in 25 per cent of cases (Fig. 16.1). The Philadelphia (Ph^1) chromosome is present in more than 90 per cent of cases. The reciprocal exchange of material between the long arms of chromosomes 9 and 22 involves translocation of the c-*abl* oncogene to chromosome 22, possibly a critical event in malignant transformation. The product of the 'fusion gene' between c-*abl* and the 'break-point cluster region' on chromosome 22 has now been identified and serves as a unique marker of CML.

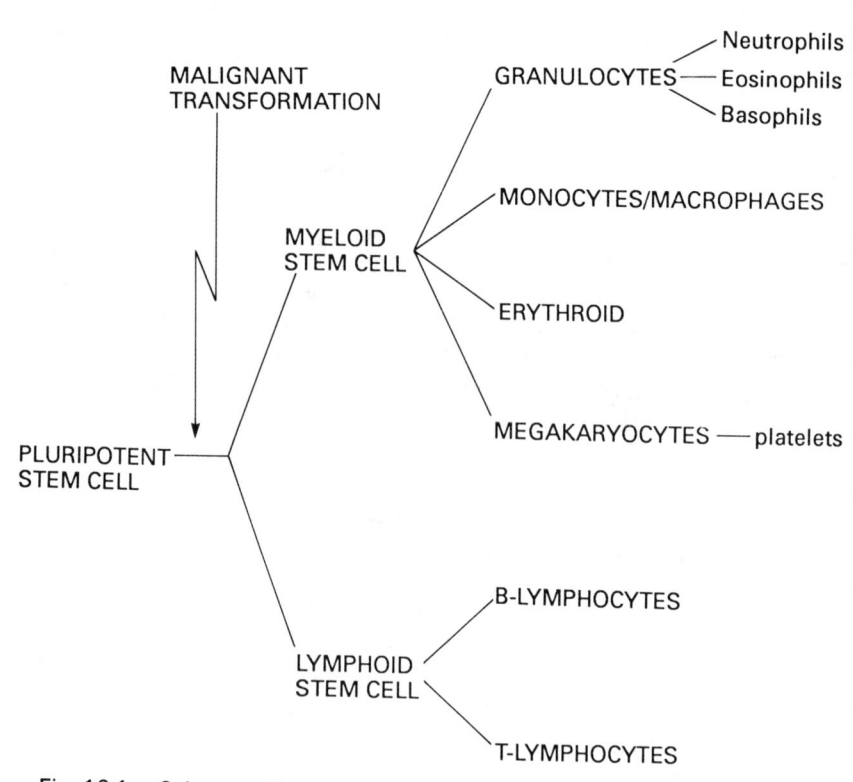

Fig. 16.1. Schema of haemopoietic differentiation from the pluripotential stem cell. With increasing differentiation, cells become 'committed' to a particular lineage. In chronic myeloid leukaemia, the malignant event affects an early stem cell. During the chronic phase, the 'thrust' of the disease involves differentiation and maturation along the myeloid line, but after transformation to the acute phase, either acute myeloid (75 per cent) or acute lymphoblastic (25 per cent) leukaemia may occur.

Symptoms and Signs

Early asymptomatic cases are occasionally diagnosed on routine blood counts. The inexorably rising white cell count is accompanied by increasing splenomegaly (first palpable at about $100 \times 10^9/1$). Massive splenomegaly often produces a sensation of abdominal fullness or pain due to splenic infarction. Moderate hepatomegaly is usual, but lymphadenopathy is rare. With advancing disease, there is prominent sweating, malaise, wasting and weight loss with a raised basal metabolic rate. Grossly elevated white cell counts ($500-1000 \times 10^9/1$) cause impaired blood flow in small vessels. Leucostasis is a medical emergency, and symptoms may include blurring of vision, epistaxis, bruising, priapism, confusion and coma. Characteristic dilatation of retinal veins and multiple retinal haemorrhages assist in diagnosis.

Investigations

The median white cell count at diagnosis is about $200 \times 10^9/1$, and progressive anaemia is seen as the leucocyte count rises. The platelet count may be normal, low or markedly increased. Examination of the blood film shows an increase in both mature and immature granulocytes with characteristic polymorph and myelocyte 'peaks' in the differential count. Basophilia and eosinophilia are common, and blast cell counts up to 10 per cent are not unusual. The bone marrow is grossly hypercellular with hyperplasia of granulocytes and megakaryocytes. Neutrophil alkaline phosphatase score is very low or zero, and serum vitamin B_{12} levels are high (increase in granulocyte-derived transcobalamins I and III). Cytogenetic analysis reveals the Ph^1 chromosome (t[9;22]) in 90 per cent of cases (*see* above). In the rare cases of 'juvenile chronic myeloid leukaemia', the Ph^1 chromosome is absent and high levels of fetal haemoglobin are seen.

Transformation to the acute phase is usually heralded by a rising blast cell count and the blood picture of acute leukaemia.

Complications

In addition to leucostasis, the chronic phase may be complicated by hyperuricaemia, gout and folate deficiency due to increased cell turnover. The acute phase is dominated by bone (and/or splenic) pain and the problems of marrow failure (bleeding and infection).

Treatment

During the chronic phase, CML is usually easily controlled by oral alkylating agents, such as busulphan. Reduction of the white cell count is accompanied by regression of hepatosplenomegaly, disappearance of systemic symptoms and return of haemoglobin to normal over several weeks. The major risk of treatment with busulphan is the unpredictable development of marrow aplasia which may be dangerously prolonged. Aggressive combination chemotherapy is more hazardous and has not proved superior to simpler treatments. Splenectomy in chronic phase also fails to improve the prognosis. In patients presenting with dangerous leucostasis, rapid reduction of the white cell count by leucopheresis on a cell-separator may be life-saving.

Intermittent courses of busulphan produce a near-normal quality of life in most patients with CML but all are fated to undergo eventual transformation to the acute phase. This is often preceded by a period when the chronic phase blood picture becomes less responsive to alkylating agents ('accelerated phase'). Transformation is commonly accompanied by the acquisition of new chromosomal abnormalities – so-called clonal evolution. About 75 per cent of patients develop an acute myeloid leukaemia which is usually refractory to conventional chemotherapy and fatal within two to three months. It is important to identify the 25 per cent who transform to acute lymphoblastic leukaemia as appropriate treatment can produce a high rate of remission and survivals of the order of 12 months.

In view of the bleak prognosis in CML, several innovative treatments have been explored. Alpha-interferon can control the leucocyte count during the chronic phase and may reduce the proportion of Ph^1-positive metaphases. Whether this will result in longer survival remains to be proven. The most hopeful innovation has been the high success rate of allogeneic bone marrow transplantation in chronic phase for the minority of patients who have a histocompatible sibling donor. The possibility of transplantation should be explored in all patients less than 50 years of age.

Prognosis

With conventional treatment, CML is an invariably fatal disease with a median survival of only 3·5 years. Five to 10 per cent of patients die within the first year, the mortality is then approximately 25 per cent per year. Philadelphia chromosome-negative CML carries a poorer prognosis. With ablative chemo- and radiotherapy followed by allogeneic bone marrow transplantation, between 50 and 75 per cent of patients may be cured. Once the acute phase has supervened, transplantation probably salvages no more than 15 per cent.

CHRONIC LYMPHOCYTIC LEUKAEMIA

Definition

Chronic lymphocytic leukaemia (CLL) is a lymphoproliferative disorder which, although usually regarded separately, belongs to the spectrum of non-Hodgkin's lymphoma (see Chapter 17).

Background

CLL is the commonest leukaemia in western countries. Its aetiology is unknown, but a familial tendency has been observed. Exposure to ionizing radiation is not implicated. CLL is largely a disease of the middle-aged and elderly, and there is a male preponderance of two or three to one.

Pathology

Small, morphologically 'mature' lymphocytes accumulate in bone marrow, lymph nodes, the reticulo-endothelial system and peripheral blood. Surface marker studies show that these cells are nearly always monoclonal B-lymphocytes at an early stage of differentiation, although rare cases of T-cell CLL are recorded.

Symptoms and Signs

The increased use of 'routine' full blood counts leads to around 25 per cent of cases presenting at an early presymptomatic stage. Common presenting symptoms include the awareness of enlarged lymph nodes and symptoms due to anaemia, e.g. tiredness, exertional dyspnoea, claudication and angina pectoris. With advancing disease, systemic symptoms such as malaise, fevers, sweats and weight loss may be prominent. Bleeding due to thrombocytopenia, and splenic or bony pain, are less common presentations. Patients with more advanced disease are immuno-deficient and bacterial lung infections are a frequent problem.

Patients usually have enlarged, rubbery, painless lymphadeno-pathy in many areas. Hepatosplenomegaly occurs with progressive disease, and infiltration of skin and other organs may occasionally be present. Leucostasis is much less common than in CML, even at extremely high white cell counts.

Investigations

The white cell count is often in the range of $50-100 \times 10^9/1$ at presentation, although modern surface marker studies allow the diagnosis to be confirmed at levels of $5.0 \times 10^9/1$ or less. An excess of small lymphocytes is present in the blood film. These cells appear fragile and are easily disrupted in spreading the blood film, producing the characteristic 'smear cells'. The lymphocytes of CLL possess only small amounts of surface immunoglobulin and typically form rosettes with mouse red cells. With progressive marrow infiltration, normocytic anaemia and thrombocytopenia occur. Both auto-immune haemolytic anaemia (positive direct antiglobulin test) and thrombocytopenia occur with increased frequency in CLL and must be differentiated from the cytopenias of marrow failure when staging the disease (Table 16.1). The degree of marrow infiltration can be accurately assessed only by trephine biopsy.

Low levels of serum immunoglobulins correlate with the defect in humoral immunity seen in advanced CLL. Up to 50 per cent of patients have a detectable serum paraprotein (with identical idiotype to the leukaemia cells) when sensitive methods are used.

Table 16.1
THE RAI STAGING OF CHRONIC LYMPHOCYTIC LEUKAEMIA

Stage	Features	Median survival (months)
0	Lymphocytosis greater than $15 \times 10^9/1$	150+
I	Lymphocytosis plus lymphadenopathy	105
II	Lymphocytosis and lymphadenopathy plus enlarged liver and spleen	71
III	Lymphocytosis and lymphadenopathy plus anaemia (haemoglobin less than 11 g/dl)	19
IV	Lymphocytosis and lymphadenopathy plus thrombocytopenia (less than $100 \times 10^9/1$)	19

Note: Anaemia and thrombocytopenia due to auto-immune destruction must be excluded.

Complications

Increased cell turnover may cause hyperuricaemia and gout. A small proportion of patients show transformation into an aggressive high grade lymphoma (Richter's syndrome) of poor prognosis. Other complications include increased risk of second malignancies (20 per cent in some studies) and membranous glomerulonephritis with nephrotic syndrome.

Staging

The most commonly used system is that of Rai (Table 16.1) which is based on a combination of clinical and haematological parameters and correlates reasonably well with increasing tumour mass and prognosis.

Treatment

Attempts at intensive curative therapy in CLL have generally been unsuccessful. As many of the patients are elderly, treatment is largely palliative in intent. Asymptomatic patients with stable disease are usually not treated, and an initial period of observation is important. Accepted criteria for treatment include progressively rising leucocyte counts with troublesome systemic symptoms or organomegaly. Auto-immune cytopenias and progressive marrow failure are also indications for therapy.

Local radiotherapy was for a long time the mainstay of treatment, and splenic irradiation may produce a generalized effect on the disease as circulating lymphocytes are depleted. Oral alkylating agents are now the most usual treatment. Low doses of oral chlorambucil given daily cause few side effects and produces a clinically beneficial reduction in leucocytosis and organomegaly in 50 to 75 per cent of cases. Intermittent (every four to six weeks) high doses of chlorambucil seem equally effective and may carry a lower risk of mutagenesis and secondary malignancy. Corticosteroids are also useful, especially as initial therapy in patients with marrow failure and to treat the complications of auto-immune haemolysis or thrombocytopenia. Long-term administration of steroids should be avoided because of the increased risk of infection and the other well-known complications, such as osteoporosis and glucose intolerance.

Conventional treatment usually produces a partial remission, and further treatment is given as needed to maintain a stable clinical condition. Immunoglobulin levels remain depressed, and susceptibility to infection persists. A more aggressive approach to achieving complete remission with combination chemotherapy produces a greater incidence of early morbidity, but preliminary evidence suggests improved survival rates in certain subgroups of patients with advanced disease.

Adjunctive treatment in CLL includes the use of allopurinol to prevent hyperuricaemia and intravenous γ-globulin to reduce infectious complications. Interferons appear of little value in CLL, although most studies to date have mainly included patients with very advanced disease.

Prognosis

The median survival according to stage in Rai's 1975 series is seen in Table 16.1. Older patients with early disease often die of unrelated illness. Infection is a prominent cause of death at all stages, and the negative effects of bone marrow failure are clearly seen.

PROLYMPHOCYTIC LEUKAEMIA

This lymphoproliferative disorder has been separated from CLL as a distinct clinical entity in recent years. The characteristic features of prolymphocytic leukaemia (PLL) include massive splenomegaly with minor or absent lymphadenopathy, prominent systemic symptoms and very high leucocyte counts (often in excess of $200 \times 10^9/1$). The 'prolymphocytes' have prominent central nucleoli and appear to represent B-lymphocytes of rather higher maturity than typical CLL. Rare cases of T-cell PLL are also described.

The prognosis is poorer than CLL, and the optimal treatment remains uncertain. Splenic irradiation or splenectomy may be helpful, and combination chemotherapy may produce remission.

HAIRY-CELL LEUKAEMIA

Definition

Hairy-cell leukaemia (synonym, leukaemic reticulo-endotheliosis) is a lymphoproliferative disorder which commonly presents with a combination of massive splenomegaly, absent lymphadenopathy, pancytopenia and characteristic circulating 'hairy cells'.

Background

Hairy-cell leukaemia is an uncommon disease of unknown aetiology, comprising less than two per cent of all leukaemias. The median age of onset is 52 years, and there is a marked male predominance of about five to one.

Pathology

Bone marrow, liver and spleen are infiltrated by mononuclear cells with long cytoplasmic projections ('hairs') which are best seen by phase-contrast microscopy. Surface marker studies confirm that in most cases the hairy cells are B-lymphocytes with a higher degree of maturation than those of CLL or PLL. A minority of cases have T-cell features.

Symptoms and Signs

The onset of disease is often insidious. Malaise, exertional dyspnoea and abdominal discomfort due to the enlarged spleen are frequent presenting symptoms. A minority present with bleeding or infective problems and systemic 'B'-symptoms are uncommon.

More than 90 per cent of patients have splenomegaly, often massive. Hepatomegaly occurs in 25 to 50 per cent but lymphadenopathy is rarely present. Occasional patients develop leukaemic skin infiltrates.

The pancytopenia is due to a combination of bone marrow failure and hypersplenism.

Investigations

Most patients present with normochromic anaemia, leucopenia and thrombocytopenia. The characteristic hairy cells are identifiable in the blood film in most patients. Neutropenia and monocytopenia are typical findings. Occasional patients develop extremely high numbers of circulating hairy cells, usually after splenectomy. Bone marrow is often inaspirable and trephine biopsy shows heavy infiltration by hairy cells and conspicuous reticulin fibrosis. The hairy cells have typical features on cytochemistry and electron microscopy, which may assist in diagnosis.

Ten to 20 per cent of patients have abnormal liver function tests at diagnosis, and a minority have a circulating paraprotein.

Differential Diagnosis

The morphology and phenotype of the mononuclear cells, and

the absence of lymphadenopathy, aids distinction from CLL. Trephine marrow biopsy excludes aplastic anaemia.

Complications

Infectious complications are extremely common and are the cause of death in 50 to 75 per cent of patients. Atypical mycobacterial infections appear to be a special problem and may reflect the severe monocytopenia. Severe vasculitic problems are a rare but well-recognized complication.

Treatment

The clinical course of hairy-cell leukaemia is highly variable, ranging from a benign course with prolonged survival to a rapidly progressive illness with death from infection or bleeding. Untreated, most patients develop a slowly increasing infiltration of the marrow and other organs with hairy cells.

Splenectomy usually causes an improvement in peripheral blood counts and splenectomized patients have been shown to have improved survival. However, at least 30 per cent of patients have progressive disease requiring other treatment. The results of intensive combination chemotherapy have been disappointing and, until recently, most patients were treated with continuous low-dose chlorambucil with variable benefit. Patients with grossly raised leucocyte counts after splenectomy could often be controlled for long periods by regular leucopheresis on a cell-separator.

The use of α-interferon has been a major breakthrough in the treatment of hairy-cell leukaemia. Up to 75 per cent of patients respond to the long-term administration of interferon with normalization of blood counts, reduction in marrow infiltration and regression of splenomegaly. Relapse usually occurs after treatment is stopped, and the optimum 'maintenance' regimen has yet to be determined. The influence of this treatment on survival is also not yet clear. Deoxycoformycin, an adenosine deaminase inhibitor, is also proving to be highly effective in hairy-cell leukaemia, and the result of long-term studies are also awaited. The exact place of these new treatments will become clearer with increasing experience.

Prognosis

With conventional treatment, the median survival in hairy-cell leukaemia is four to five years. About 10 per cent of cases have an indolent course and 30-year survival is reported. The long-term survivors tend to be older at presentation and have less prominent splenomegaly, fewer circulating hairy cells and less severe neutropenia. If symptom-free, such patients may be best left untreated until progressive disease ensues.

FURTHER READING

Gale R.P., Foon K.A. (1987). Biology of chronic lymphocytic leukaemia. *Semin. Hematol.*, **24**, 209–229.

Goldman J.M. (1986) Bone marrow transplantation for patients with chronic myeloid leukaemia. *New Engl. J. Med.*, **314**, 202–207.

Chapter Seventeen

Non-Hodgkin's Lyphomas and Hodgkin's Disease

NON-HODGKIN'S LYMPHOMAS

Definition

A non-Hodgkin's lymphoma (NHL) is the malignant (monoclonal) proliferation of B-lymphocytes, T-lymphocytes or (rarely) histiocytes. In the broadest sense, the NHLs include chronic lymphocytic leukaemias, hairy-cell leukaemia and plasma cell proliferations (Waldenström's macroglobulinaemia, myeloma), which are usually considered separately.

Background

The NHLs comprise about two per cent of all cancers. Most are of unknown aetiology, although Epstein–Barr virus is implicated in African Burkitt's lymphoma and certain lymphomas in immunodeficient patients. A specific retrovirus, HTLV-1, is associated with T-cell lymphoma/leukaemia in patients of Caribbean or Japanese origin.

Pathology

Monoclonal antibody studies show that many lymphomas correspond to recognizable stages of B- or T-lymphocyte maturation. Histological classification is complicated by the plethora of available systems and poor reproducibility of diagnosis between pathologists. Earlier systems were based purely on morphological features, whereas newer classifications incorporate knowledge of tumour immunology. The 'working formulation' of the US National Cancer Institute (Table 17.1), based on pattern of infiltration and cell type, is widely used to provide a 'common language' for pathologists. Fortunately for the physician, most classifications, whatever their complexity, categorize lymphomas into three basic groups according to their rate of clinical progression – low, intermediate or high grade.

Symptoms and Signs

The non-Hodgkin's lymphomas are among the most heterogeneous of diseases in presentation. The classical presentation is

Table 17.1
CLASSIFICATION OF NON-HODGKIN'S LYMPHOMA
(NATIONAL CANCER INSTITUTE WORKING FORMULATION)

Low grade
Small lymphocytic (phenotypically identical to chronic lymphocytic leukaemia)
Follicular, predominantly small cleaved cell
Follicular, mixed small cleaved and large cell

Intermediate grade
Follicular, predominantly large cell
Diffuse, small cleaved cell
Diffuse, mixed small and large cell
Diffuse, large cell

High grade
Large cell, immunoblastic
Lymphoblastic
Small, non-cleaved cell

Miscellaneous
Mycosis fungoides
Histiocytic
Extramedullary plasmacytoma
Unclassifiable
Other

with enlargement of lymph nodes at one or more sites, commonly with hepatosplenomegaly. Symptoms may arise from local nodal enlargement, e.g. respiratory embarrassment or superior vena caval obstruction due to mediastinal disease (especially in T-cell NHL) or abdominal swelling, ascites or lower limb oedema with bulky intra-abdominal (para-aortic, iliac, mesenteric) disease. Extensive bone marrow involvement may cause clinical symptoms due to anaemia, neutropenia or thrombocytopenia. Central nervous system involvement may occur, especially in intermediate or high grade disease. Patients with coeliac disease may develop multifocal aggressive gut lymphomas which are now known to be derived from T-lymphocytes. Cutaneous lymphomas (e.g. mycosis fungoides or Sézary's syndrome) are also usually of T-cell origin, and characteristic cells with 'convoluted' nuclei may be seen.

It is important to elicit a history of 'B-symptoms' (Table 17.2) which usually indicate disseminated disease.

Table 17.2
ANN ARBOR STAGING SYSTEM

Stage
I	Nodal involvement within one region
IE	Single extralymphatic organ or site
II	Nodal involvement of two or more regions limited by diaphragm
IIE	Localized extranodal site and nodal involvement within one or more regions bounded by the diaphragm
III	Nodal involvement of regions above and below the diaphragm
IIIE	As III but with localized extranodal disease
IIIS	As III plus splenic involvement
IV	Disseminated involvement of one or more extralymphatic organs, with or without lymph node involvement

Systemic symptoms
'A' documents the absence and 'B' the presence of
    Unexplained fever above 38 °C
    Night sweats
    Unexplained weight loss of more than 10% in six months

Investigations

These are directed to confirming the diagnosis and establishing the extent (stage) of disease (Table 17.2). Diagnosis usually requires biopsy of appropriate nodal or other involved tissue. Histological examination is often augmented by histochemical or immunological studies. Examination of the blood film may reveal circulating lymphoma cells, especially in low grade 'follicular' lymphomas. Aspiration and trephine biopsy of bone marrow commonly reveals focal involvement by follicular lymphoma (of no prognostic significance), whereas marrow involvement in the higher grades is less common, usually diffuse and of more serious import. Anatomical staging usually includes chest radiography, abdominal ultrasound examination and computerized tomography. Lymphangiography, isotope liver and spleen or bone scans, and radiological studies of gut or skeleton may be indicated in particular cases. Staging laparotomy is not indicated.

Differential Diagnosis

Differential diagnosis is usually from other malignant neoplasms or Hodgkin's disease.

Complications

These include recurrent infection predisposed by low immunoglobulin levels and impaired humoral immunity, hyperuricaemia and gout due to increased cell turnover, and the additional problems of hyperkalaemia and hyperphosphataemia in the 'tumour lysis syndrome' which may occur after chemotherapy of aggressive high grade lymphomas. Auto-immune haemolytic anaemia or thrombocytopenia may also be seen.

Treatment and Progress of Disease

Accurate diagnosis and staging is essential so that appropriate treatment can be tailored to the precise grade and stage of disease.

Low grade lymphomas

Low grade lymphomas usually occur in the middle-aged or elderly. About 10–15 per cent have truly localized (Stage I or II) disease, which may be cured by local radiotherapy. It is important to note that perhaps 50 per cent of patients with Stage III or IV disease pursue an indolent course, and specific treatment can be safely delayed until clinical problems or cosmetically unacceptable disease occurs. Combination chemotherapy is hazardous and not curative in this group; however, relatively non-toxic treatment with oral alkylating agents (usually chlorambucil) may produce good clinical control. Prolonged treatment with low dose chlorambucil should be avoided because of the risk of secondary leukaemia. Alpha-interferon is active in low grade NHL, but its use is yet to be defined. Many patients eventually show progression to a more aggressive histology and respond poorly to further treatment.

Intermediate and high grade lymphomas

These tend to occur in a younger age group, usually pursue an aggressive course and are rapidly fatal if untreated. Stage I disease is relatively uncommon, and good results have been reported with both radiotherapy and combination chemotherapy (more appropriate in younger patients). Most patients present with Stage III or IV disease and need combination chemotherapy. Recent results with intensive (often weekly) multidrug regimens report a complete remission rate of 60–80 per cent and long-term survival (cure?) in 30–40 per cent of patients. Such results are obtained at the expense of significant toxicity and the need for high quality supportive care similar to that required for patients with acute leukaemia. Central nervous system prophylaxis with cranial irradiation and intrathecal methotrexate should be considered in patients with lymphoblastic lymphoma. High-dose chemoradiotherapy followed by infusion of stored autologous bone marrow is showing encouraging results in patients with early and chemoresponsive disease but produces little benefit in those with relapsed or refractory lymphoma.

Cutaneous lymphomas

Cutaneous lymphomas are usually of T-cell (commonly 'T-helper') origin. They may remain indolent and confined to skin for many years and respond to local treatment (radiotherapy, 'PUVA' or topical alkylating agents). Once a more aggressive phase with nodal and marrow involvement ensues, the prognosis is poor with conventional chemotherapy, although recent encouraging results with α-interferon have been reported.

HODGKIN'S DISEASE

Definition

Hodgkin's disease (HD) is a malignant disorder which primarily involves lymphoid tissue. Compared with the non-Hodgkin's lymphomas, HD is less often widely disseminated at presentation and tends to spread in an orderly fashion to contiguous lymph node groups.

Background

The aetiology of HD remains unknown, although epidemiological 'clustering' of cases has raised speculation as to an infective (viral?) origin. It is commonest in the third to fifth decades of life, and there is a male preponderance.

Pathology

The cell type of HD remains uncertain, although recent studies suggest a lymphoid (possibly T-cell) rather than a 'histiocyte' origin. Characteristic Sternberg–Reed cells usually form a minority of cells present in the involved node, and a variety of histological patterns is recognized (Table 17.3). In general, lymphocyte-predominant HD has the most favourable prognosis and lymphocyte-depleted histology the worst.

Symptoms and Signs

Almost any tissue or organ may be affected, but most patients present with painless enlargement of lymph nodes, commonly in

Table 17.3
RYE CLASSIFICATION OF HODGKIN'S DISEASE

Histology	Approximate frequency (%)
Lymphocyte-predominant	10–15
Nodular sclerosing	20–50
Mixed cellularity	20–40
Lymphocyte-depleted	5–15

the neck. Mediastinal involvement may cause superior vena caval obstruction or bronchial compression. Intra-abdominal disease may be represented by hepatosplenomegaly or palpable para-aortic nodes and marrow involvement may lead to pancytopenia or painful sclerotic bone lesions. Intracerebral, spinal or epidural involvement may occasionally be seen and present with signs of a space-occupying lesion or spinal cord compression. The presence of 'B-symptoms' (Table 17.2) usually implies advanced stage disease. Alcohol-induced pain at the site of nodal disease is an unusual but characteristic feature of HD, and generalized pruritus may also occur.

Investigations

Diagnosis must be confirmed by a lymph node or tissue biopsy. Secondary anaemia is common in advanced HD, and a peripheral blood oesinophilia may occur. Marrow involvement is much less common than in NHLs and is most readily diagnosed by trephine biopsy. HD is staged in a similar manner to the NHLs (Table 17.2), using a combination of radiology, ultrasound, computerized tomography and scintiscanning. As the treatment modality may be critically dependent on accurate staging, it has been common practice to perform a staging laparotomy with diagnostic splenectomy and liver biopsy in patients with apparently localized disease suitable for radiotherapy. Thirty per cent of patients with clinical Stage I or II disease have occult intra-abdominal disease present at laparotomy.

Complications

In addition to the local anatomical problems caused by tumour masses and infiltration, patients with advanced HD have impaired cell-mediated immunity and susceptibility to opportunistic infection.

Differential Diagnosis

This is usually from NHL or other malignant diseases, although tuberculosis and sarcoidosis may be considered in patients with mediastinal adenopathy and/or pulmonary infiltration.

Treatment

Localized Stage I or II HD is usually treated with radiotherapy alone. The area irradiated is designed to cover contiguous nodal areas on the same side of the diaphragm, e.g. the 'mantle' and 'inverted-Y' fields for disease above and below the diaphragm, respectively. Planning of the field and radiation dosage attempts to minimize the risk to radiosensitive tisses, such as lungs, kidney, gonads and spinal cord. Stage IIIA disease may be treated with total nodal irradiation, but there is an increasing trend to use chemotherapy in this setting.

Stage IIIB and IV disease is treated with cyclical combination chemotherapy. Following the success of the 'MOPP' regimen (mustine, vincristine, prednisolone, procarbazine), many newer combinations have been studied in an attempt to increase efficacy and reduce toxicity. Alternating cycles of 'non cross-reactive' combinations are now often used in an attempt to reduce acquired tumour cell drug resistance. It is conventional to give two or three cycles of chemotherapy after complete remission is achieved (averages 6–8 cycles), and radiotherapy to areas of bulky disease may follow or be 'sandwiched' in the regimen. These combinations produce significant and predictable toxicity, including myelosuppression, nausea and vomiting, alopecia, neurotoxicity and impaired gonadal function; therefore, good supportive facilities and expert staff are essential. Maintenance chemotherapy does not improve duration of remission or survival.

Prognosis

About 20 per cent of patients with Stage I and II disease relapse within five years of radiotherapy, but a majority of these respond as well to chemotherapy as do previously untreated patients.

Complete remission rates of 60–80 per cent are now commonly reported in patients with advanced HD treated with combination chemotherapy. About 50 per cent of the responders remain in long-term remission and may be cured. Relapse is most common in the first three years after treatment but has been recorded at up to 15 years. Poor prognostic factors include male sex, lymphocyte-depleted histology, bulky mediastinal disease, older age and B-symptoms. Children with HD have an excellent prognosis with chemotherapy, with up to 94 per cent five-year survival reported. 'Salvage' chemotherapy after relapse may produce a further remission in 50 per cent of patients, but long-term survival is uncommon. There have been recent encouraging reports of the efficacy of high-dose 'ablative' chemo- and radiotherapy followed by autologous bone marrow transplantation in these patients. Male sterility is usual after combination chemotherapy for HD, and pretreatment cryopreservation of sperm should be offered. Recovery of ovarian function is more common (especially in younger women), but a premature menopause is the rule. Use of the contraceptive pill during chemotherapy may have a protective effect on ovarian function.

The risk of secondary leukaemia after successful treatment for HD is increasingly recognized. Alkylating agents are particularly mutagenic and patients treated with both chemo- and radiotherapy are at the highest risk (*see* Chapter 20). Radiotherapy alone seems to be non-leukaemogenic.

FURTHER READING

McElwain T.J., Lister T.A., eds. (1987). The lymphomas. *Clin. Haematol.*, **1**(1), 1–269.

Chapter Eighteen

Myeloma and the Immunocytomas

INTRODUCTION

Humoral immunity is mediated by antibodies (immunoglobulins) produced by cells of the B-lymphocyte system. Antibody molecules are composed of two 'light' and two 'heavy' chains, and five classes of immunoglobulin (Ig) are recognized (Table 18.1). Normally, in response to an antigenic stimulus, many 'clones' of B-lymphocytes are stimulated to proliferate and differentiate. The end result is the production of a range of similar, but not identical, antibodies which recognizes determinants present on the antigen (a 'polyclonal' response). Any single B-cell clone can produce Ig with only κ- or λ-light chains ('light chain restriction'), and therefore the usual polyclonal response (both κ- and λ-chains present, usually in a ratio of about 2:1) can readily be distinguished from a 'monoclonal' (derived from a single cell) antibody response in which all the Ig molecules possess light chains of the same class. Such monoclonal immunoglobulins are referred to as 'paraproteins' or M-proteins and are of significance

Table 18.1
CLASSIFICATION AND PROPERTIES OF IMMUNOGLOBULINS

Class	Heavy chain	Molecular weight (kd)
G	Gamma (γ)	150
A	Alpha (α)	160–320 (dimers)
M	Mu (μ)	900 (pentamers)
D	Delta (δ)	185
E	Epsilon (ε)	200

in a number of haematological diseases. Paraproteins may also be recognized by the formation of a narrow 'band' on a serum protein electrophoretic strip, reflecting the identical physical properties of the Ig molecules. Free light chains may be detected in urine as 'Bence–Jones protein' in certain pathological states.

MONOCLONAL GAMMOPATHY OF UNDETERMINED SIGNIFICANCE

Definition

This condition is defined by the presence of a monoclonal protein in people with no evidence of myelomatosis or similar disorder. The label monoclonal gammopathy of undetermined significance (MGUS) is preferred to 'benign paraproteinaemia' as it is impossible to predict whether any individual case will eventually develop myelomatosis or macroglobulinaemia.

Investigations and Prognosis

Various population studies have shown an incidence of MGUS in the population ranging from one per cent of people over 25 years of age to three per cent of those over 70 years. As protein electrophoresis is increasingly carried out in routine 'biochemical profiles', incidental paraproteins are being seen more commonly in clinical practice. In a long-term study of 241 cases at the Mayo Clinic, the actuarial incidence of myeloma was 17 per cent at 10 years and 34 per cent at 15 years from diagnosis. Such studies suggest that patients with low risk of progression to myeloma usually have normal concentrations of haemoglobin and serum albumin, less than five per cent bone marrow plasma cells, a low paraprotein concentration, no Bence–Jones proteinuria, no osteolytic lesions and no evidence of progression on extended follow-up. No single parameter can identify the risk of progression in the individual patient. An association with MGUS has been claimed for many diseases, but large studies with age-matched controls are usually lacking. No treatment is indicated for MGUS, and most patients are simply followed on an annual basis, although there is no evidence that the presymptomatic treatment of myelomatosis is beneficial. A significant proportion of patients with IgM paraproteins will eventually show evidence of non-Hodgkin's lymphomata.

MYELOMATOSIS

Definition

This is a monoclonal proliferation of mature, usually antibody-secreting, plasma cells. The incidence is approximately two per 100 000, it is rare before the fourth decade and the mean age of onset is 63 years. Apart from the rare 'solitary plasmacytoma of bone', myelomatosis is a disseminated disease at the time of presentation.

Diagnosis

Diagnosis is usually based on the presence of at least two of the following criteria: more than 20 per cent plasma cells in bone marrow smears; presence of a paraprotein in blood urine; lytic bone lesions. Approximately 50 per cent of patients have an IgG paraprotein in serum, 25 per cent have IgA, two per cent have IgD and less than one per cent are 'non-secretory'. Seventeen per cent of patients have light chain only myelomas, but Bence–Jones proteinuria is found in 70 per cent of those who can produce complete Ig molecules.

Symptoms and Signs

The clinical problems in myeloma are due to combinations of bone marrow infiltration and failure, skeletal damage, renal impairment, hypercalcaemia, infection or hyperviscosity.

Bone pain is the commonest presenting symptom, often worse at night and exacerbated by exercise. Pathological fractures may occur through osteolytic lesions in the long bones, ribs or vertebral bodies (with the risk of compression paraplegia). Less common presentations relate to symptoms of uraemia or anaemia in the absence of bone pain, infection (bacterial pneumonia, shingles) or hypercalcaemia (usually coincident with renal failure and extensive skeletal disease). The concentration and physical properties of some paraproteins (especially the dimers of IgA) may lead to the 'hyperviscosity syndrome' with progressive confusion, lethargy, purpura, mucous membrane haemorrhage and visual disturbance with a characteristic retinopathy. Minor hepatomegaly is common in myelomatosis, but lymphadenopathy and splenomegaly are unusual.

Investigations

The blood count commonly reveals a normochromic anaemia. Leucopenia and thrombocytopenia may reflect the degree of marrow infiltration. When high paraprotein concentrations are present, the red cells often form characteristic 'rouleaux' in the blood film. Such cases also have a raised erythrocyte sedimentation rate (ESR) or plasma viscosity. Bone marrow infiltration with plasma cells is often patchy, and a trephine biopsy gives more complete information than the aspirate alone.

The combination of clinical suspicion and characteristic blood changes leads to electrophoresis of serum and urine to detect a paraprotein or free light chains. These can be identified and quantitated. Biochemical assessment of renal function and serum calcium are mandatory.

Conventional radiology is more sensitive than isotope scanning to demonstrate bony lesions. A full skeletal survey will reveal characteristic lytic lesions in about 60 per cent of patients. Lesions may be single or multiple, are characteristically round and well-circumscribed and most prevalent in the axial skeleton. Generalized osteoporosis is also seen, and myeloma cells are known to release an 'osteoclast activating factor'.

Treatment and Prognosis

Many parameters have prognostic significance in patients with myelomatosis. Various staging systems based on combinations of clinical and biochemical measurements have been proposed. More recently, simpler measures, such as the pretreatment haemoglobin and blood urea or serum β_2-microglobulin have been shown to provide equally powerful information.

There is no curative treatment, and therapy is aimed at arresting progress of the disease and relieving symptoms. Early cases with no clinical problems should not be treated – survival is not prolonged, and treatment merely hastens the onset of drug-resistance and the risk of secondary leukaemia.

The simple measures of ensuring a high (three litres per day) oral fluid intake and early, vigorous treatment of infection have done much to reduce the early mortality in myeloma. Radiotherapy may be used to produce rapid control and pain relief at areas of localized bony disease. The oral alkylating agent melphalan (1-phenyl alanine mustard) produces an objective response in about 50 per cent of patients. Response may be slow, and maximal improvement may take several months. The majority of responders show a reduction in tumour mass and paraprotein level and then enter a so-called 'plateau phase' in which further treatment is probably unhelpful. Prolonged treatment leads to acquired drug resistance and carries a high risk of producing secondary myelodysplasia and leukaemia. Combination chemotherapy is more toxic, but recent studies suggest that higher response rates may be translated into longer survival. Once relapse occurs, about one third of patients will achieve a short response to combination chemotherapy, but clinical benefit is often poor. The median survival in most series remains only 30 to 40 months. Hypercalcaemia and renal failure at presentation may respond well to intravenous saline and steroids, and haemodialysis may be useful in selected patients. Agents such as calcitonin, diphosphonates and mithramycin may also be helpful. Chronic renal failure in the context of stable disease is not a contra-indication to long-term dialysis. Recent heroic treatments such as bone marrow transplantation and ultra-high dose melphalan perhaps offer the prospect of cure or long-term survival in a small minority of younger patients. Recent evidence suggests that α-interferon may have a role in prolonging plateau phase and survival. Interest has revived in the use of higher dose corticosteroids in patients with relapsed or refractory disease, in whom response rates equivalent to many combination chemotherapy regimens may be obtained with significantly less toxicity and improved quality of life.

WALDENSTRÖM'S MACROGLOBULINAEMIA

Definition

This is a lymphoproliferative disorder involving so-called 'lymphoplasmacytoid' cells, which are immediately below mature plasma cells in the B-cell maturation pathway. Many of the clinical features of this disease are intermediate between those of classical lymphomas (lymphadenopathy, hepatosplenomegaly) and myelomatosis (paraproteinaemia, bone marrow infiltration). The characteristic 'macroglobulin' is an IgM paraprotein which forms pentamers of high molecular weight (900 kd) and results in large increases in plasma viscosity.

Symptoms and Signs

This is largely a disease of the elderly and is rare before the fourth decade. Patients with classical macroglobulinaemia present with symptoms and signs of hyperviscosity (*see* above) and may have little clinically detectable tumour. Others may have a 'lymphomatous' presentation, with lymphadenopathy and hepatosplenomegaly and clinically insignificant levels of macroglobulin. Bone marrow failure with pancytopenia is more common in the lymphomatous form. Skeletal involvement is rare. Patients are immuno-incompetent and have increased susceptibility to infection.

Investigations

Presence of a paraprotein may be suspected by the combination of a very high ESR (or plasma viscosity) and rouleaux of red cells on the blood film. Lymphoplasmacytoid cells may appear in the blood, marrow and affected lymph nodes. The IgM will be detected on serum protein electrophoresis and identified by immunofixation.

Treatment and Prognosis

This is often a slowly evolving disorder, and no curative therapy is available. Asymptomatic patients may simply be observed and may remain well for many years. The dangerous hyperviscosity syndrome responds well to plasma exchange (usually performed on an automated cell-separator), as the paraprotein is largely intravascular. Removal of relatively small amounts of paraprotein can produce a dramatic fall in plasma viscosity. The rate of IgM production may be low enough to allow some patients to be managed by intermittent plasma exchange alone.

Patients with progressive lymphomatous disease, especially with marrow failure, require chemotherapy to reduce tumour mass. Alkylating agents such as chlorambucil and cyclophosphamide, often in combination with prednisolone, may produce good palliation. After many years, patients often become refractory to alkylating agents, but response to more aggressive regimens is usually poor in this largely elderly group. There appears to be a higher than expected incidence of other malignant diseases in patients with Waldenström's macroglobulinaemia.

AMYLOIDOSIS

In this group of disorders, an abnormal fibrillary protein is deposited, locally or systemically in extracellular sites. Amyloid fibrils are arranged in characteristic 'β-pleated sheets', which are relatively resistant to proteolytic digestion. In histological sections, amyloid fibrils take up the dye Congo red and exhibit apple-green birefringence in polarized light. Amyloidosis can be classified according to the major protein from which the fibrils are derived, and a variety of clinical syndromes are distinguished (Table 18.2).

Systemic Amyloidosis

Amyloidosis due to excessive or abnormal production of immunoglobulin light chains (AL amyloid) is seen in up to 15 per cent of cases of myelomatosis. In 'primary amyloidosis', there is no evidence of systemic myeloma, but most patients have a detectable serum paraprotein or Bence–Jones proteinuria, especially if sensitive techniques are used. Although amyloid can be

Table 18.2
CLASSIFICATION OF AMYLOIDOSIS

Syndrome	Amyloid fibril	Serum protein
Systemic amyloidosis		
Immunocytoma (e.g. myeloma, primary amyloid)	AL	Immunoglobulin light chain
Reactive (chronic infection, malignancy)	AA	Serum amyloid-A protein
Heredofamilial syndromes (e.g. familial Mediterranean fever)	AA	Serum amyloid-A protein
Localized amyloidosis		
Senile cardiac amyloid	ASc_1	Pre-albumin
Immunocyte-derived	AL	Immunoglobulin light chain
Haemodialysis-associated	β_2-M	β_2-microglobulin

deposited in any tissue or organ, there is a predilection for 'mesenchymal' tissues and symptoms may include macroglossia, peripheral neuritis (rare in reactive amyloidosis), carpal tunnel syndrome and restrictive cardiomyopathy.

Reactive amyloidosis (AA) is derived from the acute phase reactant protein, serum amyloid-A protein. Examples of predisposing diseases are seen in Table 18.3. There is a predilection for infiltration of kidney, spleen and liver, but any tissue can be involved. Clinical presentation commonly includes nephrotic syndrome or hepatosplenomegaly.

Familial Mediterranean fever is the commonest of the heredofamilial amyloidoses (AA). In this autosomal, recessively inherited disease, patients usually have sporadic attacks of abdominal pain, vomiting, fever and arthritis, accompanied by the development of progressive systemic amyloidosis with prominent renal involvement.

Table 18.3
CAUSES OF REACTIVE AMYLOIDOSIS (AA)

Chronic/recurrent infection	Chronic inflammation	Malignant disease
Tuberculosis	Rheumatoid disease	Hodgkin's disease
Bronchiectasis	Ankylosing spondylitis	Renal carcinoma (rarely other carcinomas)
Osteomyelitis	Behçet's disease	
Cystic fibrosis	Systemic lupus	
	Dermatomyositis	

Localized Amyloidosis

Local amyloid deposits are found in the brain of many elderly people and in the neurofibrillary tangles characteristic of Alzheimer's disease. Cardiac amyloid deposition increases with age ('senile cardiac amyloidosis', ASc_1) and rarely causes clinical symptoms. Localized cutaneous amyloidosis is fairly common, particularly in the form of pruritic papules on exterior surfaces.

Haemodialysis-Associated Amyloid

Carpal tunnel syndrome and other problems of local amyloid deposition in patients on chronic haemodialysis are now known to be due to aggregates of β-microglobulin, a low molecular weight protein, which is inadequately cleared by many dialysis membranes.

Diagnosis

A high index of clinical suspicion is necessary in view of the protean manifestation of amyloidosis. Renal amyloid is typified by non-selective proteinuria, bilateral enlargement and progressive renal failure (especially in AA amyloidosis). Cardiac involvement is common in all forms of systemic amyloidosis, classically producing biventricular failure with a normal heart size on chest

X-ray. Echocardiography shows thickening of myocardium. Respiratory involvement is usually seen in AL amyloid. Gastrointestinal involvement is common in all forms and may produce dysphagia, severe diarrhoea, ulceration, haemorrhage or malabsorption. The neuropathy (usually AL amyloid) is predominantly sensory, and palpable nerve enlargement may be present. Definitive diagnosis is by biopsy of the affected organ, although rectal biopsy or aspiration of subcutaneous fat is positive in about 75 per cent of cases of systemic amyloidosis. Examination of serum and urine for monoclonal proteins is usual, and marrow biopsy helps to exclude myelomatosis.

Treatment

No medical treatment is known to reverse amyloid deposition, although there are convincing reports of reduction in proteinuria in AL amyloid treated with cytotoxic agents. Control of the underlying disease may delay the progression of reactive systemic amyloidosis. Colchicine reduces the frequency of acute attacks in familial Mediterranean fever and may inhibit amyloid formation, but appears of little use in other forms of amyloidosis. Haemodialysis or peritoneal dialysis may prolong survival in those with renal involvement, and renal transplantation may be successful. Dialysis-associated amyloid is reduced in incidence by the use of membranes which enhance the clearance of β_2-microglobulin.

Prognosis

Systemic amyloidosis is usually fatal, death generally occurring from renal or cardiac disease. Mean survival in AL amyloidosis ranges from 12 months (non-myeloma group) to only six months in those with myeloma. Survival is longer in the reactive forms, depending on the progression of underlying disease as well as the effects of amyloid deposition.

FURTHER READING

Delamore I.W., ed. (1986). *Multiple Myeloma and Other Paraproteins*. Edinburgh and London: Churchill Livingstone.

Chapter Nineteen

Polycythaemia

DEFINITION

Polycythaemia (synonym, erythrocytosis) is defined as an increase in the levels of haemoglobin, red cell count and haematocrit in the peripheral blood. Although this picture may reflect a true increase in red cell mass, many cases seen in clinical practice have an apparent erythrocytosis due to a reduction in plasma volume ('relative' or 'spurious' polycythaemia, sometimes known as Gaisböck's syndrome). Consequently, the measurement of red cell mass and plasma volume allows cases to be categorized as 'true' or 'relative' polycythaemia. The former group can be classified as 'primary' (polycythaemia vera) or 'secondary' to an underlying stimulus (Table 19.1).

DIAGNOSIS

History and Physical Examination

These are the essential first steps and will guide the intelligent selection of laboratory investigations.

Polycythaemia vera

Polycythaemia vera is largely a disease of the middle-aged and elderly and is more common in males. It is a malignant haematological disorder belonging to the spectrum of myeloproliferative syndromes (Fig. 19.1). The common symptoms and signs reflect the increase in blood volume and whole-blood viscosity (of which haematocrit is the major determinant), and changes in biochemistry and metabolic rate due to myeloproliferation. Patients

Table 19.1
CLASSIFICATION AND CAUSES OF POLYCYTHAEMIA

Primary
　Polycythaemia vera (synonym, primary proliferative polycythaemia)

Secondary
　Physiological increase in erythropoietin (hypoxia)
　　Respiratory failure
　　Cardiovascular disease
　　Congenital heart disease
　　High altitude
　　High affinity haemoglobins
　　Chronic methaemoglobinaemia
　　Heavy smoking

　Miscellaneous
　　Renal disease (simple cysts, polycystic disease, hypernephroma, vascular disease)
　　Uterine fibromyomas
　　Adrenal tumours
　　Hepatocellular carcinoma
　　Cerebellar haemangioblastoma

Relative
　'Stress' polycythaemia
　Gaisböck's syndrome
　Dehydration or acute plasma loss (e.g. burns)

often present with lassitude, headaches, visual disturbance, weight loss or night sweats. Pruritis, often exacerbated by hot baths, is a frequent complaint. The course of the untreated disease is dominated by thrombo-embolic, peripheral vascular and bleeding complications, which may be presenting features. Unusual thrombic events, such as mesenteric or hepatic venous thrombosis, are particularly associated with polycythaemia vera. Increased cell turnover and hyperuricaemia may be reflected in acute gout or tophaceous disease.

On examination, patients usually have a plethoric complexion and conjunctival suffusion. Moderate splenomegaly is found in more than 50 per cent of patients, and hepatomegaly is common.

Essential thrombocythaemia⇌Polycythaemia vera⇌Myelofibrosis

(Intermediate forms of these discrete syndromes are commonly seen; patients with long-standing polycythaemia vera tend to develop features of myelofibrosis. Transformation to acute myeloid leukaemia may be a terminal event.)

Fig. 19.1. Myeloproliferative disorders.

Secondary polycythaemia

The clinical picture will reflect the symptoms and signs of the underlying disease (Table 19.1). Hypoxia in patients with respiratory or cardiac disease may cause central cyanosis (e.g. the 'blue bloater' with chronic airways disease) and clubbing of the extremities. A family history of polycythaemia might suggest the inheritance of a high oxygen affinity haemoglobin variant (e.g. haemoglobin Chesapeake) or congenital methaemoglobinaemia. Polycythaemia is a physiological response to living at high altitude. Heavy smoking is associated with high levels of carboxyhaemoglobin, which may produce tissue hypoxia and polycythaemia.

The presence of an abdominal mass (other than splenomegaly) may point to the diagnosis of renal or uterine tumours, and signs of cerebellar dysfunction or raised intracranial pressure to a rare cerebellar haemangioblastoma.

Relative polycythaemia

This condition is at least 10 times as common in clinical practice as polycythaemia vera. Acute changes in plasma volume may occur in patients with severe burns or enteritis. The aetiology of 'stress polycythaemia' or Gaisböck's syndrome is unknown. Patients tend to be overweight, plethoric and hypertensive. There may be a relationship to the use of diuretics or cigarette smoking. Without special investigations, it may be difficult to distinguish from early polycythaemia vera. However, as with secondary polycythaemia, thrombotic and haemorrhagic complications are much less common and the hypermetabolic symptoms of primary polycythaemia are absent.

Investigations and Laboratory Data

Although higher levels of haematocrit (above 0·55) suggest the presence of true polycythaemia, measurement of red cell mass (^{51}Cr-labelling of erythrocytes) and plasma volume (^{131}I-labelling of albumin) are necessary to exclude relative polycythaemia reliably.

Primary polycythaemia

In addition to the diagnostic increases in haemoglobin, haematocrit and red cell count, patients often have a reduced mean corpuscular volume (MCV) due to increased iron utilization by the expanded erythroid compartment. Some degree of generalized myeloproliferation is usual, and there is a variable increase in white cell and platelet counts. Increase in basophils and eosinophils may be seen. Advanced cases with myelofibrotic features may show 'tear-drop poikilocytes' in the blood film and become progressively anaemic. Bone marrow aspiration and trephine biopsy show a hypercellular marrow with reduced fat spaces, and an increase in red cell precursors, granulocytes, megakaryocytes and, often, reticulin. The ability of erythroid precursors to proliferate in culture independently of erythropoietin stimulation may be specific for primary polycythaemia and other myeloproliferative disorders.

Biochemical abnormalities include raised levels of vitamin B_{12} (due to raised levels of transcobalamins I and III from myeloid cells) and uric acid. Folate deficiency may occur because of increased cell turnover. Despite these features, the diagnosis of primary polycythaemia may be a process of exclusion.

Secondary polycythaemia

Hypoxia in respiratory or cardiac disease can be confirmed by measurement of arterial oxygen saturation. Special investigations, such as lung function tests and radiography, are dictated by clinical findings. The miscellaneous causes may require investigations such as ultrasound, computerized tomography scanning or intravenous pyelography. Measurement of $P_{50}O_2$ will exclude a high affinity haemoglobin. Morphology of blood and bone marrow is normal except for the increase in erythropoietic activity.

Relative polycythaemia

Relative polycythaemia is associated with normal blood and bone marrow morphology in the absence of coexisting disorders. The polycythaemia is usually only mild or moderate (haematocrit rarely above 0·6).

Management

Polycythaemia vera

Treatment is directed at controlling blood viscosity and the symptoms related to myeloproliferation. Patients with mild disease may be treated by venesection alone. It may be optimal to maintain the haematocrit below 0·45, but regular venesection may produce severe iron deficiency and does not control other features of the disease. Myelosuppressive therapy may be given as intermittent (e.g. 6–9 monthly) intravenous injections of radiophosphorus (^{32}P – a β-emitter which localizes in bone) or as oral alkylating agents (e.g. chlorambucil or busulphan). ^{32}P is convenient to administer, requires less rigorous monitoring of blood counts, and is especially useful in the elderly. The large American Polycythaemia Vera Study Group trial (Berk et al., 1986) showed that patients treated with oral busulphan had longer survival and fewer thrombotic complications than comparable patients managed by venesection or ^{32}P. However, this group has also shown that the chronic administration of chlorambucil produces an unacceptably high (approximately 13 times) risk of acute myeloid leukaemia, and a similar, albeit delayed, incidence of secondary leukaemia is now evident in the group tested with ^{32}P. An acceptable compromise may be to manage younger patients by venesection alone, if possible. If myelosuppressive therapy is necessary, the antimetabolite hydroxyurea may be a less leukaemogenic alternative. About two per cent of patients treated with venesection alone develop acute leukaemia.

Adjunctive treatments include prevention of gout by prophylactic allopurinol (xanthine oxidase inhibitor) and avoidance of folic acid deficiency. Pruritis may be an intractable problem, often responding poorly to myelosuppressive therapy or symptomatic treatment with antihistamines.

Secondary polycythaemia

Correction of the underlying cause (if possible) is the primary aim of treatment. The value of venesection in patients with a 'physiological' increase in haematocrit (e.g. due to hypoxia) is debatable. However, it is undeniable that some patients with respiratory or cardiac disease may obtain relief of symptoms such as headache, and improved cerebral blood flow after venesection has been shown in certain studies. The prognosis is that of the underlying disease.

Relative polycythaemia

Relative polycythaemia may often be corrected by control of risk factors such as obesity, smoking, hypertension and diuretic therapy. The value of venesection is once again debatable, but a few patients do report relief of minor symptoms such as headache.

PROGNOSIS

The median survival for 431 patients in the Polycythaemia Vera Study Group trial (Berk *et al.*, 1986) is 11·8 years for patients treated with ^{32}P, 8·9 years for chlorambucil and 13·9 years for venesection. In the first four years of study, the venesected group had, however, a high incidence of thrombotic complications. Beyond five years, there is a disproportionate incidence of deaths from cancer and leukaemia in patients treated with standard myelosuppressive therapy. Whether the use of hydroxyurea will produce an acceptable 'compromise', with a lower incidence of both thrombosis and leukaemia, remains to be seen.

REFERENCES

Anon. (1987). Pseudopolycythaemia. *Lancet*, **ii**, 603–604.
Berk P.D., Goldberg J.D., Donovan P.B., et al. (1986). Therapeutic recommendations in polycythaemia vera based on Polycythaemia Vera Study Group protocols. *Semin. Haematol.*, **23**, 132–143.

Chapter Twenty

Myelodysplasia and Secondary Leukaemia

PRIMARY MYELODYSPLASIA

Definition

The primary myelodysplastic syndromes (MDS) are a group of disorders characterized by peripheral blood cytopenias, ineffective haemopoiesis and a hypercellular bone marrow. There is a variable tendency to progress to acute myeloid leukaemia, and synonyms include 'preleukaemia' and 'smouldering leukaemia'.

Background and Pathology

These are largely disorders of the elderly and arise from the malignant transformation of a primitive bone marrow stem cell whose progeny include cells of the myeloid series (granulocytes, erythrocytes and megakaryocytes). At least 50 per cent of these patients have non-random chromosome abnormalities, and the majority of marrow cells belong to the malignant clone at the time of diagnosis. Although five distinct syndromes are recognizable by peripheral blood and bone marrow studies (French/American/British classification), these diseases fall into two main groups with regard to prognosis and risk of leukaemic transformation (Table 20.1). The spectrum of clinical and laboratory features is wide and tends to progress with time; therefore, individual patients may be difficult to classify. A substantial proportion of patients in all groups never develop acute leukaemia and loaded terms such as 'preleukaemia' are perhaps best abandoned.

Table 20.1
CLASSIFICATION AND PROGNOSIS OF MYELODYSPLASTIC SYNDROMES

Syndrome	Blast cells (%) Blood	Marrow	Progression to leukaemia (%)	Median survival (months)
RARS	<1	<5	10	70
RA	<1	<5	15	65
CMML	<1	5–20	30	10
RAEB	<5	5–20	40	10
RAEB-T	>5	20–30	60	5

RARS = refractory anaemia with ring sideroblasts; RA = refractory anaemia; CMML = chronic myelomonocytic leukaemia; RAEB = refractory anaemia with excess blasts; RAEB-T = RAEB in transformation.

Symptoms and Signs

Presenting symptoms and signs usually result from the consequences of bone marrow failure or qualitative abnormalities of platelets and neutrophils. However, many patients are first diagnosed on an incidental blood examination whilst still asymptomatic. Weakness due to anaemia, infection and haemorrhage are common presenting symptoms. On examination, pallor, purpura and petechiae may be present; lymphadenopathy is rare and hepatosplenomegaly is largely seen in those with chronic myelomonocytic leukaemia (CMML), in whom leukaemic skin infiltrates may also occur.

Investigations

Morphological examination of blood and marrow is the cornerstone of diagnosis. Ninety per cent of patients are anaemic at presentation, typically with macrocytosis of red cells. Fifty per cent of patients are neutropenic, and common abnormalities include a reduction in neutrophil granules or nuclear hyposegmentation (Pelger-Hüet abnormality). Patients with CMML have, by definition, more than $1.0 \times 10^9/l$ peripheral blood monocytes. Although thrombocytopenia is also common, occasional patients (with the 5q$^-$ chromosome abnormality) may present with thrombocytosis.

Bone marrow aspiration and biopsy is essential and usually demonstrates a hypercellular marrow in striking contrast to the peripheral cytopenias (ineffective haemopoiesis). Red cell abnormalities may include megaloblastic features, multinuclearity and increased deposition of iron in mitochondria (ring sideroblasts). White cell precursors may show abnormal granularity and a relative increase in immature forms. The presence of distinctive mononuclear ('micro') megakaryocytes may assist in diagnosis.

Cytogenetic analysis reveals non-random chromosome abnormalities in 50 per cent of patients, and these are more frequent in the highly 'preleukaemic' group, i.e. CMML, refractory anaemia with excess blasts, (RAEB) and RAEB in transformation (RAEB-T). Development of new chromosome abnormalities commonly precedes leukaemic transformation.

Vitamin B_{12} levels are normal, but increased marrow cell turnover may lead to folate deficiency or hyperuricaemia. Increased levels of lysozyme in blood and urine are a feature of CMML. Acquired red cell membrane abnormalities may include loss or weakening of the A blood group antigen or a positive Ham's test (increased sensitivity to complement as in paroxysmal nocturnal haemoglobinuria). Qualitative defects in neutrophil and platelet function are common and may cause infection and bleeding despite near-normal concentrations.

Differential Diagnosis

The main distinctions to be made are from megaloblastic anaemia (vitamin B_{12} and folate levels) in refractory anaemia (RA) and secondary sideroblastic anaemia in refractory anaemia with ring sideroblasts (RARS) (Table 20.2). Absence of the characteristic Philadelphia chromosome helps to distinguish CMML from chronic granulocytic leukaemia. RAEB and RAEB-T are distinguished from overt acute myeloid leukaemia by the lower percentage of marrow blast cells and observation of the rate of disease progression.

Complications

In patients with RA and RARS, the main clinical problems are usually anaemia and the complications of frequent red cell

Table 20.2
SIDEROBLASTIC ANAEMIA

Congenital
  Sex-linked (partial) recessive – rare

Acquired
  Primary: Refractory anaemia with ring sideroblasts (ring sideroblasts may also be present in smaller numbers in other MDS)

  Secondary: Pyridoxine deficiency   ⎱ Vitamin B_6
             Antituberculous chemotherapy ⎰ antagonism

             Lead poisoning   ⎫
             Erythropoietic porphyria   ⎬ Haem synthesis
             Chloramphenicol   ⎪ disturbance
             Alcohol (?)   ⎭

             Rheumatoid arthritis   ⎫
             Carcinoma   ⎪
             Haemolytic anaemia   ⎬ Miscellaneous
             Megaloblastic anaemia   ⎪
             Myxoedema   ⎭

transfusion. Leukaemic transformation is relatively uncommon in this group. Recurrent infection and bleeding tends to dominate the clinical picture in RAEB, RAEB-T and CMML, and progression to acute leukaemia is common. Patients with MDS appear to have a higher than average incidence of other malignant diseases.

Treatment

No specific curative treatment is possible for most patients with MDS; therefore, great care must be taken to maintain the quality of life. Supportive therapy is the mainstay of treatment before leukaemic transformation. Red cell transfusions should be given as clinically needed. The longer natural history of RA and RARS may necessitate regular transfusion over a period of years, and chelation therapy with desferrioxamine could be considered to prevent the hepatic, cardiac and endocrine damage of iron overload. White cell-depleted blood will reduce the frequency and severity of febrile transfusion reactions. Platelet transfusions are usually reserved for specific bleeding episodes or to cover surgical procedures. Early, vigorous treatment of infective episodes with broad spectrum antibiotics is vital in these immunocompromised patients. Attention to oral and perianal hygiene, and administration of topical antiseptic and antifungal agents, may be helpful. Prophylactic folate supplements and allopurinol are commonly prescribed to reduce the complications of high marrow cell turnover.

A period of observation is important in all patients with MDS to judge the rate of progression of disease before considering specific chemotherapy. Patients with stable or slowly progressive disease are best served by supportive care alone. Aggressive combination chemotherapy is poorly tolerated in these elderly patients, prolonged marrow aplasia is common and complete remissions are generally brief. Once overt acute myeloid leukaemia has developed, the results of standard chemotherapy are dismal; 30 to 40 per cent complete remission rates with few patients achieving long-term survival. Such results have led to interest in other forms of treatment. In vitro studies suggest that agents such as low-dose cytosine arabinoside, 1,25-dihydroxy vitamin D_3 ($1,25(OH)_2D_3$) and 13-*cis* retinoic acid can induce differentiation and maturation in the dysplastic clone of cells. Clinical results have been less encouraging and side effects are prominent; however, exploration of this mode of treatment continues. Occasional patients with RARS show a reticulocytosis and reduced transfusion requirement with high-dose oral pyridoxine. The rare young patient (less than 30 years) with MDS may be cured by ablative chemoradiotherapy and allogeneic bone marrow transplantation.

Prognosis

The risk of progression to acute leukaemia and median survival of each main MDS variant is seen in Table 20.1. Patients with RA or RARS commonly die of unrelated causes, whereas those with CMML, RAEB or RAEB-T usually die of infection, bleeding or leukaemic transformation.

SECONDARY MYELODYSPLASIA AND LEUKAEMIA

Definition

Secondary leukaemia has long been recognized as a hazard of exposure to industrial mutagens such as benzene. As more patients with malignant diseases experience long-term survival after successful chemo- and radiotherapy, cases of therapy-induced MDS and acute leukaemia are being seen with increasing frequency.

Background and Pathology

The therapeutic agents most commonly implicated are alkylating agents, such as chlorambucil and cyclophosphamide, whereas antimetabolites and anthracyclines appear to carry a much lower risk. Combined therapy with alkylating agents and radiotherapy seems especially dangerous, but radiotherapy alone is of doubtful significance. The risk of secondary leukaemia in patients treated successfully for Hodgkin's disease or non-Hodgkin's lymphomas is at least five per cent with a median onset five years after treatment. Long-term survivors of myeloma have a 10 to 20 per cent incidence of MDS/leukaemia, and cases are being reported in patients receiving adjuvant chemotherapy for solid tumours such as breast or colon. The use of cytotoxic agents in non-malignant diseases is clearly hazardous.

Symptoms and Signs

Most cases are first noticed by abnormalities in routine follow-up blood counts. As the disease progresses, the symptoms and signs are identical to patients with RAEB or RAEB-T.

Investigations

The usual first abnormality on the blood film is unexplained red cell macrocytosis, followed by increasing pancytopenia. Marrow examination shows changes similar to primary MDS.

Prognosis

The 'preleukaemia' phase in these patients is generally less than one year. Once overt acute myeloid (commonly myelomonocytic) leukaemia develops, only 20 per cent respond to standard chemotherapy and mean survival is only five months. Allogeneic marrow transplantation may be considered in younger patients. Much effort is now being put into devising effective but less leukaemogenic drug regimens for the treatment of malignant disease.

FURTHER READING

Bennett J.M., Catovsky D., Daniel, M.T., et al. (1982). Proposals for the classification of the myelodysplastic syndromes. *Brit. J. Haematol.*, **51**, 189–199.

Hamblin T.J., Oscier D.G. (1987). The myelodysplastic syndrome – a practical guide. *Haematol. Oncol.*, **5**, 19–34.

Chapter Twenty One
Myelofibrosis

The term myelofibrosis denotes an increase of collagen in the marrow, which may also be accompanied by new bone formation (osteosclerosis). In addition, there may be blood formation in other organs, especially the liver and spleen (extramedullary haemopoiesis). Myelofibrosis may be primary or secondary to a number of other conditions or toxic insults to the marrow (Table 21.1).

PRIMARY MYELOFIBROSIS

Definition

Primary myelofibrosis is a member of the spectrum of myeloproliferative disorders (*see* Chapter 19), which also includes polycythaemia vera and essential thrombocythaemia. It may arise

Table 21.1
CAUSES OF MYELOFIBROSIS

1. Primary myelofibrosis

2. Secondary:
    Carcinoma
    Hodgkin's disease
    Leukaemia (especially megakaryocytic)
    Tuberculosis
    Systemic lupus erythematosus
    Benzene
    Fluorine
    Radiation

de novo or as an end stage of the myeloproliferative process. Progressive fibrosis and osteosclerosis of the marrow is accompanied by extramedullary haemopoiesis in liver and spleen, marrow failure and hypersplenism.

Background

The aetiology is unknown. Patients between 40 and 70 years of age are most commonly affected, and the sex incidence is equal.

Pathology

In common with other myeloproliferative disorders, this is a clonal disease arising from a primitive haemopoietic stem cell. Proliferation of megakaryocytes may induce secondary proliferation of fibroblasts, possibly in response to 'platelet-derived growth factor'. There is unequivocal evidence that the proliferating fibroblasts in the bone marrow do not belong to the malignant clone.

Symptoms and Signs

Presentation may be with the insidious onset of weakness due to anaemia, sweats, fever and weight loss. Splenic enlargement often causes abdominal discomfort or painful splenic infarction. Bleeding from thrombocytopenia and gout due to hyperuricaemia may also be presenting symptoms. There is a significantly increased risk of peptic ulcer disease.

Gross splenomegaly is the cardinal physical sign, the spleen often extending into the right iliac fossa. Mild to moderate hepatomegaly is usual, but lymphadenopathy is rare. Purpura may be present in patients with thrombocytopenia, and signs of portal hypertension are common in advanced cases.

Investigations

The characteristic blood picture is of a 'leuco-erythroblastic anaemia' with circulating immature granulocytes and nucleated red blood cells. Tear-drop shaped red cells are typically seen. The anaemia is usually normocytic unless folate deficiency is also present. An increase in white cell count is common and may occasionally simulate chronic myeloid leukaemia. However, the leucocyte count rarely exceeds $100 \times 10^9/1$, and the Philadelphia chromosome is absent. The platelet count may be high, normal or low at presentation but usually falls in the course of the disease.

Bone marrow aspiration is often unsuccessful ('dry tap'), and trephine biopsy is essential for diagnosis. There is a variable increase in reticulin and collagen, often with osteosclerosis and islands of haemopoietic tissue with increased megakaryocyte numbers. It is not usually considered necessary to demonstrate extramedullary haemopoiesis by liver biopsy or splenic aspiration. Radiological evidence of osteosclerosis may be present, especially in the pelvis, spine and upper femora.

The massive splenomegaly causes both pooling and destruction of red cells and platelets and an increase in plasma volume with dilutional anaemia. Increased serum lactate dehydrogenase may reflect increased erythroid activity.

Treatment

The disease usually runs a fairly chronic course with progressive splenomegaly and bone marrow failure. Treatment is largely symptomatic, with red cell transfusion as clinically indicated and vigorous treatment of intercurrent infection. Exclusion of folate deficiency and prevention of hyperuricaemia with allopurinol are important adjunctive measures. Painful splenic enlargement, especially with a rising white cell count, may be helped by oral busulphan or hydroxyurea. Splenic irradiation is usually only of temporary benefit. Splenectomy may be hazardous and does not improve survival; however, it may improve the quality of life in patients with recurrent infarction, severe thrombocytopenia or excessive transfusion requirements. Splenectomy is occasionally followed by massive liver enlargement or severe thrombocytosis. In general, thrombocytopenia is the most difficult problem to treat; steroids are usually unhelpful, and long-term platelet transfusion support is impractical.

Prognosis

Infection, bleeding, thrombosis and portal hypertension are the common causes of death. The mean survival is four or five years from diagnosis, but survival of 20 years or more has been reported in rare instances. Ten per cent of patients develop acute myeloid leukaemia which is refractory to chemotherapy and usually rapidly fatal.

ACUTE MYELOFIBROSIS

Acute myelofibrosis (synonym, malignant myelosclerosis) is now thought to represent a form of acute megakaryoblastic leukaemia. The clinical picture is dominated by infection, bleeding and systemic symptoms. There is pancytopenia with small numbers of circulating blast cells and myelofibrosis without prominent hepatosplenomegaly. Blast cells in the marrow are shown to be of megakaryocytic origin by marker studies and electron microscopy. Response to chemotherapy may be poor and survival is generally short.

FURTHER READING

Kelsey P.R., Geary C.G. (1987). Management of idiopathic myelofibrosis. *Clin. Lab. Haematol.*, **9**, 1–12.

Chapter Twenty Two

Aplastic Anaemia

DEFINITION

In aplastic anaemia, there is a pancytopenia resulting from a marrow of reduced cellularity without infiltration, fibrosis or deficiency of folic acid or vitamin B_{12}.

BACKGROUND

Aetiology

The causes of aplasia are summarized in Table 22.1. Transient hypoplasia is expected after conventional doses of chemotherapeutic drugs and radiotherapy, but higher doses (as used in marrow transplantation) destroy the stem cells and no recovery follows. High doses of radiotherapy alone to a local area of marrow will cause permanent local aplasia, but marrow elsewhere compensates for the loss.

In about half the cases of prolonged and serious aplasia, the cause cannot be established. The commonest identifiable causes are drugs and hepatitis. Certain drugs can cause an idiosyncratic and unpredictable aplasia in a small percentage of people (e.g. chloramphenicol affects one in 30 000 patients). Many patients developing aplasia have been on multiple drugs; the link with any particular drug may be impossible to establish and some innocent drugs may be blamed. The better established drugs are shown in Table 22.2. Non-B hepatitis may precede aplasia by about six weeks, particularly in young males, and the prognosis in these patients is poor. In susceptible individuals, chemicals at home and work may cause aplasia, and these include paints with solvents

Table 22.1
CAUSES OF APLASTIC ANAEMIA

Idiopathic
   About 60% of cases

Drugs
   Chemotherapy
   Idiosyncratic

Radiotherapy
   High doses to areas of active marrow

Chemicals
   Benzene and solvents, e.g. for paints, glues, dyes

Virus infection
   Hepatitis–A virus (delayed and severe aplasia)
   Parvovirus and Epstein–Barr virus (transient effect)

Haematological
   Paroxysmal nocturnal haemoglobinuria, PNH
   Pre-acute lymphoblastic leukaemia in children

Inherited
   Fanconi's anaemia.

Pregnancy

Table 22.2
DRUGS DEFINITELY KNOWN TO CAUSE APLASTIC ANAEMIA

Antibiotics	Chloramphenicol (1/20 000 patients)
	Sulphonamides
Anti-inflammatory	Phenylbutazone (1/100 000)
	Oxybutazone
	Gold salts
	Amidopyrine
Others	Chlorpropamide
	Chlorpromazine
	Potassium perchlorate
	Organic arsenicals
	Mepacrine

and benzenes, glues for model making, and hair dyes (in the past, when anilines were used).

Very rare causes include paroxysmal nocturnal haemoglobinuria (PNH), which may present with aplasia rather than haemolysis, and Fanconi's anaemia.

Transient hypoplasia of the marrow, with recovery within a few weeks, is common after virus infections (e.g. Epstein–Barr virus and type B19 parvovirus) and may cause lowering of the platelet and leucocyte counts; anaemia is not usually seen, but in haemolytic anaemias it may develop rapidly because of the shortened red cell survival.

Incidence

In Europe, the incidence is about one in 100 000 of the population per year, but in the Far East, with more hepatitis and greater use of chloramphenicol, the incidence is much greater.

Pathogenesis

Simple depletion of the pluripotential stem cells is probably the **main** cause of aplasia in about half of the patients, as identical twin studies show that the aplasia can be corrected by simple infusion of marrow cells. In others, immunosuppression is needed before the infusion, implying that immune mechanisms against the stem cell are active. The success of transplantation in treatment is against the concept of a hostile marrow micro-environment leading to aplasia.

SYMPTOMS AND SIGNS

The presentation is with bleeding problems, infections and anaemia. Lymphadenopathy is not seen, hepatomegaly is rare and splenomegaly (found in only 10 per cent) is only slight.

The platelet count usually falls gradually, and patients commonly present with a history of a few weeks of skin and mucosal haemorrhage. Skin rashes from purpura of the skin, nose-bleeds and gum bleeding are common presentations, but haematuria, menorrhagia, gastro-intestinal bleeding and problems from fundal and central nervous system haemorrhages may be the cause of presentation. Less frequently, patients present with infections, particularly of the throat and respiratory tract.

Fanconi's anaemia is an autosomal recessive disorder which usually presents with symptoms of aplastic anaemia at about the age of five years. Associated skin and skeletal abnormalities are usually found, with shortness of stature, pigmented skin, hypoplasia of the radius and thumb and loss of carpal bones or syndactyly, microcephaly, deafness and renal abnormalities all fairly common.

The important distinction between mild aplastic anaemia, which requires supportive treatment, and severe aplastic anaemia (SAA), which requires more radical treatment, is based on the laboratory findings.

INVESTIGATIONS

Pancytopenia is found at presentation in most patients, but those showing initial cytopenia in only one or two cell lines usually develop pancytopenia within a few months. Thrombocytopenia is found in the vast majority of patients, with counts under $30 \times 10^9/l$ in over 70 per cent. The leucocyte count may be within the normal range, but the neutrophil count is usually reduced. Lymphocytes and monocytes may be normal or low.

Anaemia may be marked. The red cells are usually dysplastic and the mean corpuscular volume (MCV) is normal or raised a little, but vitamin B_{12} and folate levels are normal. In anaemia with a normally functioning marrow, the reticulocyte count usually rises in response to the anaemia, but this is unusual in aplastic anaemia where even the absolute reticulocyte count is low ($<25 \times 10^9/l$) in two thirds of cases. A high reticulocyte count for the haemoglobin level raises the possibility of a diagnosis of PNH.

Few immature cells (less than five per cent erythroblasts or myelocytes) are found, which contrasts with the blood film appearance in leukaemias, myelodysplasia or malignant infiltration of the marrow. The erythrocyte sedimentation rate is frequently raised, reflecting the anaemia, but the plasma viscosity is normal. Haemoglobin F levels may be raised, particularly in children.

Attempts at marrow aspiration are often unsuccessful, but may reveal empty particles. Trephine biopsy is essential. This shows widespread hypoplasia, but on occasions there are islands of activity, particularly erythroid, and repeat biopsy may be needed. An increase in lymphocytes is suggestive of an immune origin. An increase in blast cells suggests leukaemia. Cytogenetic studies in Fanconi's anaemia show chromosomal fragility, and this is greatly increased after incubation with cyclophosphamide.

Further tests are not usually needed to establish a diagnosis of aplastic anaemia, but may be helpful in establishing the aetiology, e.g. for recent hepatitis or viral infection and for PNH.

COMPLICATIONS

Abnormal clones of cells may appear later in the course of the disease. For example, PNH, with a clone of red cells very sensitive to lysis by complement, may develop, typically causing dark urine in the morning from haemoglobinuria. A more serious, but rare, example is the development of acute myeloid leukaemia, which is a particularly common complication in Fanconi's anaemia.

A worrying complication is the development of antibodies to platelets, rendering patients refractory to further platelet transfusions.

PROGNOSIS

Prognosis and treatment options are influenced by the severity of aplasia. In SAA (Table 22.3), the platelet count is $< 20 \times 10^9/1$ with neutrophils $< 0.5 \times 10^9/1$ and reticulocytes $< 20 \times 10^9/1$, and the marrow trephine shows < 30 per cent myeloid cells; in SAA, the median survival with full supportive care is under three months, compared with about 15 months for less severe cases.

Table 22.3
DEFINITION OF SEVERE APLASTIC ANAEMIA

Platelet count	$< 20 \times 10^9/1$
Neutrophil count	$< 0.5 \times 10^9/1$
Reticulocyte count	$< 10 \times 10^9/1$
Bone marrow	$> 70\%$ non-myeloid cells

With modern immunosuppressive treatment or marrow transplantation, the outlook is greatly improved, with long-term survival for over 50 per cent of patients.

TREATMENT

Supportive care for bleeding and infective problems is of the utmost importance in aplastic anaemia and should be undertaken by a specialist team, since patients who can be kept alive may make a complete recovery (even without specific treatment) many months or even years after diagnosis.

Patients with mild aplasia and only minor clinical problems are treated with supportive therapy alone.

In aplastic anaemia with bleeding or infective problems, supportive therapy alone is insufficient, and active attempts to revive the marrow should be made using either immunosuppression with antilymphocyte globulin (ALG) or marrow transplantation (from a HLA-matched sibling, or possibly from a matched unrelated donor). The choice will depend on the severity of the disease, the age of the patient and the availability of a donor.

In young patients with SAA, the treatment of choice is transplantation, and the management should be discussed with a marrow transplant team as soon as the diagnosis is suspected, with a view to early transplantation if a suitable HLA-matched sibling donor can be found. Results show a greater than 60 per cent cure rate and are best in young patients who have not been sensitized by multiple transfusions. Delays in referral may lead to death before transplantation can be arranged.

Immunosuppression using antilymphocyte globulin (ALG), prepared from horse or rabbit, acts by suppressing any immune mechanism which may be impairing stem cell growth. Side effects are common, particularly on the first day, and include anaphylactic reactions, headache, vomiting and further depression of the platelet count with bleeding. Care with administration is essential, and the reactions can be minimized by steroids and pethidine; platelet transfusions may be needed. Nearly half of the patients develop serum sickness within two weeks. Any responses are normally seen within two months of a course of treatment, and although recovery may not be complete, the rise in counts may be sufficient to improve the clinical problem. If the response is inadequate, some practitioners attempt a second course using ALG (from a different animal source) or antithymocyte globulin.

ALG is most effective in mild aplastic anaemia, but is less good in SAA or in young children. Overall, ALG therapy results in clinical improvement in over 50 per cent, but complete remission in far fewer. It has been the treatment of choice in all patients with clinically troublesome aplasia who do not meet the above criteria for sibling transplantation.

Patients with very severe neutropenia ($<0.2 \times 10^9/1$) and children under 10 years old in general show a poor response to ALG, and so when no matched sibling donor can be found (in patients under 45 years), some centres are exploring transplantation using matched unrelated donors (MUD). This technique has also been used where ALG treatment has failed. Currently, it is sometimes difficult to find suitable donors and to find them sufficiently rapidly. With the newer techniques of matching by DNA analysis, and with the building up of larger donor pools, the situation will improve. Additional problems are those of rejection and graft-*versus*-host disease (*see* Chapter 15), which are more marked with MUD transplants, but the field is one of rapid development.

Hormonal drugs designed to stimulate the marrow have been widely used in the past, but are of limited use. A few patients, particularly with mild aplasia, may show undoubted improvement in erythropoiesis after up to three months on oxymethalone or other androgens. The value of combinations of these drugs with ALG is currently being explored. Cyclosporin, which inhibits T-lymphocytes, is also undergoing clinical trials, but the list of drugs used in the past in attempts to improve aplastic anaemia is long.

The spontaneous recovery of some patients makes assessment of treatment difficult, and the rarity and severity of aplastic anaemia makes it desirable that patients should be managed by teams registering their data with international studies, so that advances can continue to be recognized.

PURE RED CELL APLASIA AND MARROW FAILURE AFFECTING SINGLE CELL LINES

On rare occasions, marrow failure may be confined to a single cell line, and this will result in either pure red cell aplasia, neutro-

Table 22.4
CAUSES OF RED CELL APLASIA

Congenital
    Diamond–Blackfan syndrome

Acquired
    Drugs, e.g. azathioprine, penicillamine, chlorpropamide
    Virus, e.g. parvovirus
    Associated with immune disorders
    Idiopathic (50% have a thymoma)

penia, or thrombocytopenia. Of these disorders, red cell aplasia is the most common (Table 22.4).

Diamond–Blackfan syndrome refers to an autosomal recessive disorder presenting at birth, or shortly after, with anaemia, profound reticulocytopenia and skeletal abnormalities, such as a triphalangeal thumb. Early treatment with intermittent steroids is usually indicated and may be required long-term. Regular transfusions, preferably with filtered or processed red cells and chelation, are often needed, and when the spleen is enlarged, splenectomy may help.

In older patients, red cell aplasia may be transient (often related to drugs or virus infection) or chronic (usually associated with immune disorders or idiopathic). Red cell aplasia secondary to drug therapy usually responds to stopping or even reducing the drug, and azathioprine after renal transplantation is now a well-recognized cause. In the idiopathic variety, a thymoma can be demonstrated (by standard and lateral chest X-ray, tomography or computerized tomography scans) in about half of the patients and may be associated with myasthenia gravis. However, thymectomy cures the red cell aplasia in only about 20 per cent of patients. Successful treatment regimens for red cell aplasia have included steroids, cyclophosphamide and splenectomy.

FURTHER READING

Champlin R.E., Feig S.A., Sparkes R.S., Gale R.P. (1984). Bone marrow transplantation from identical twins in the treatment of aplastic anaemia: implication for the pathogenesis of the disease. *Br. J. Haematol.*, **56**, 455–463.

Geary C.J., ed. (1979). *Aplastic Anaemia*. London: Baillière Tindall.

Chapter Twenty Three

Thrombosis

Thrombosis may occur in either the arterial or venous circulation. Abnormalities of the vessel wall, reduced blood flow and/or altered activity of platelets and fibrinolytic or coagulation factors (Virchow's triad) may contribute to its development. When considering pathophysiology and treatment, it is convenient to separate thrombotic events occurring in the venous and arterial circulations, although it is recognized that a degree of overlap occurs. An arterial thrombus develops in a fast flowing system in association with a damaged vessel wall. The thrombus primarily contains platelets, with other blood constituents and fibrin strands being present as secondary features. A venous thrombus develops in a slow flow system; no morphological abnormalities of the vessel wall are apparent. The thrombus consists largely of a dense fibrin mesh with trapped blood cells in a proportion that is normally present in blood.

The concept of hypercoagulability, i.e. a situation in which an abnormality of the blood can be detected which identifies an individual as being at risk for thrombotic events, has been much sought after. Attempts to recognize such individuals have largely been unsuccessful, and one cannot accurately predict which patients will develop thrombotic disease. However, there are groups of patients who do appear to have an increased tendency to develop thrombotic attacks. By measuring certain individual proteins (*see* below) which participate in the coagulation and fibrinolytic pathways, such groups of patients can be identified, although it should be stressed that many of these will not subsequently develop overt thrombotic events.

PREDISPOSING FACTORS TO VENOUS THROMBOTIC DISEASE

Secondary Causes (Table 23.1)

Venous thrombosis occurs typically in situations associated with venous stasis, e.g. postoperatively, and this explains the predilection for thrombi to occur in the low pressure venous system of the lower limbs. Stasis is not sufficient to produce a thrombus, and changes in the coagulation/fibrinolytic systems and vessel wall are probably essential co-factors.

An increased tendency to thrombosis occurs in pregnancy and those taking combined oral contraceptive agents. In pregnancy, an increase in coagulation factors, coupled with reduced fibrinolytic activity (especially apparent in the third trimester), would suggest that an increased potential for fibrin formation is present, and this is supported by the presence of fibrin deposits in the spiral arteries of the placenta. Likewise, the combined oral contraceptive agents produce similar changes in the coagulation/fibrinolytic pathways, with increased levels of circulating coagulation factors and reduced fibrinolytic activity. Preparations containing lower doses of oestrogens are associated with a reduced incidence of thrombosis.

Myeloproliferative syndromes, especially polycythaemia vera and essential thrombocythaemia, are associated with an increased tendency to thrombosis. Thrombosis may occur in unusual ana-

Table 23.1
SECONDARY CAUSES OF THROMBOSIS

Postoperative or prolonged recumbency
Obesity
Heart failure
Pregnancy
Oral contraceptives
Myeloproliferative diseases
Malignant disease
Drugs, e.g. heparin, L-asparaginase
Paroxysmal nocturnal haemoglobinuria
Lupus anticoagulant
Nephrotic syndrome
Behçet's syndrome

tomical sites, such as the splenic, hepatic and portal veins. In polycythaemia vera, the risk of thrombosis is closely associated with an increase in whole blood viscosity, and this can be significantly reduced by maintaining the packed cell volume below 0·45. In essential thrombocythaemia, qualitative abnormalities of platelet function, producing an increased responsiveness to aggregating agents in vitro, may be important. In this disease, digital ischaemia secondary to microvascular platelet aggregation may occur and can be treated effectively by an antiplatelet agent such as aspirin. In paroxysmal nocturnal haemoglobinuria, a membrane defect is present resulting in platelets which are highly sensitive to the lytic effects of complement. It is thought that complement binding may result in platelet aggregation and thrombosis.

The lupus anticoagulant, an antibody reacting with certain phospholipid-dependent coagulation reactions, is now known to occur in a variety of different clinical situations other than systemic lupus erythematosus (Table 23.2), including apparently normal healthy individuals. The presence of this inhibitor is often associated with false positive syphilis serology. It is associated, not with a haemorrhagic tendency, but with a thrombotic one. Why this is so is unclear, but this inhibitor has been demonstrated to reduce prostacyclin formation/release from vascular endothelial cells. Venous and arterial thromboses have also been described in patients with antibodies to cardiolipin.

Patients with advanced malignant disease have an increased tendency to thromboses (Trousseau's syndrome), and these may occur in unusual sites, e.g. recurrent superficial phlebitis in the upper limbs. Such events may antedate the finding of a malignancy. The reasons for a thrombotic tendency to occur in such patients are multiple, and some of the more obvious include immobilization of very ill patients and a higher incidence of

Table 23.2
LUPUS INHIBITOR AND CLINICAL ASSOCIATIONS

Systemic lupus erythematosus (SLE)
Normal, apparently healthy individuals
Auto-immune diseases other than SLE
Malignant disease
Paraprotein disorders
Immune thrombocytopenia

surgery in this group. In addition, high platelet counts, increased levels of coagulation factors and reduced fibrinolytic activity, which can be demonstrated in many patients, may be contributory. A recently recognized phenomenon is the presence in many cancer patients of chronic intravascular activation of coagulation. Intravascular activation of coagulation could promote clot formation. The activating stimulus appears to be certain tumour cells which contain a procoagulant material capable of activating the coagulation cascade locally. Furthermore, tumour cells may activate monocytes either directly or through a T-lymphocyte-mediated response. Activated monocytes contain procoagulant material on the surface membrane.

Heparin may be associated paradoxically with both venous and arterial thromboses. This is frequently preceded by thrombocytopenia which results from a heparin-induced immune reaction. The result of this is intravascular platelet aggregate formation which, in some patients, is sufficient to produce occlusive arterial thrombotic disease. Thrombocytopenia usually develops 7–14 days following the commencement of heparin therapy and is independent of the type of heparin used, dose or route of administration.

L-asparaginase, a cytotoxic agent used in the treatment of leukaemia, is associated with thrombotic events which may be secondary to its potential for reducing circulating antithrombin III (AT III) and protein C levels. Hyperviscosity syndrome and Behçet's syndrome may be complicated by recurrent thromboses. Thrombosis in patients with nephrotic syndrome may be related to an excessive urinary loss of coagulant inhibitory proteins such as AT III.

Primary Causes (Table 23.3)

Hereditary deficiencies of coagulation and fibrinolytic proteins and, more importantly, of coagulant inhibitory enzymes such as AT III and protein C may occur. The identification of quantitative or qualitative abnormalities identifies groups of patients who appear to be at risk of thrombosis. It is likely that many patients who have been subject to recurrent thrombotic events have (as a contributory factor at least) a specific enzyme defect.

Primary thrombotic disorders should be suspected in:

Table 23.3
PRIMARY CAUSES OF THROMBOSIS

Antithrombin III deficiency
Protein C deficiency
Protein S deficiency
Dysfibrinogenaemia
Dysplasminogenaemia
Plasminogen activator deficiency

1. Young patients who have no secondary cause to explain a thrombotic attack
2. Patients with recurrent venous thromboses
3. Patients with a family history of thrombosis.

The majority of people with hereditary protein deficiencies are asymptomatic and do not develop thrombotic attacks. Frequently, however, the addition of a secondary cause precipitates a thrombosis.

AT III interrupts the coagulation cascade by inhibiting thrombin activity, and AT III deficiency is the most commonly recognized defect. This is typically inherited in an autosomal dominant fashion. Thrombotic attacks occur for the first time during the second and third decades of life. Because adequate levels of AT III are required for heparin activity, acute thrombotic attacks may require treatment with AT III concentrates in addition to heparin.

Protein C is a vitamin K-dependent protein which acts by inhibiting the activity of factors V and VIII in the coagulation pathway. It also increases the activity of the fibrinolytic system. Protein S is also a vitamin K-dependent protein which acts as a co-factor for the anticoagulant activity of protein C.

Abnormalities of the fibrinolytic system, such as qualitative and quantitative defects of plasminogen and reduced quantities of plasminogen activator released from vascular endothelial cells, may increase the tendency to thrombotic attacks. Recently, an inhibitor of plasminogen activator, tissue plasminogen activator inhibitor (TPAI), has been described. This protein inhibits fibrinolysis. Patients with high levels of TPAI and associated thrombotic attacks have been described. Such abnormalities of the fibrinolytic system, with an overall reduction in fibrinolytic activity, may predispose an individual to thrombotic attacks by the impairment of fibrin digestion. Patients with a dysfibrinogenaemia, a qualitative defect of fibrinogen, may rarely be subject to thrombosis. This occurs because of an inherent resistance of fibrin to plasmin digestion.

It is important to recognize the inherited protein deficiencies in patients as appropriate counselling may be given. Family studies are then indicated, and life-long treatment with anticoagulants may be necessary. Such patients must take care to avoid the secondary causes of thrombosis.

FURTHER READING

De Swiet M. (1985). Thromboembolism. *Clinics in Haematology*, **14**(3), 643–661.
Rodgers G.M., Shuman M.A. (1986). Congenital thrombotic disorders. *Am. J. Haemat.*, **21**, 419–430.
Schafer A.I. (1985). The hypercoagulable states. *Ann. Int. Med.*, **102**, 814–828.

Chapter Twenty Four
Anticoagulant Therapy

Anticoagulant drugs are used prophylactically or to treat a current thrombotic episode. The drugs fall into five categories: oral anticoagulants, heparin, ancrod, fibrinolytic agents and drugs that interfere with platelet function.

ORAL ANTICOAGULANTS

Warfarin, a water soluble derivative of coumaric acid, is the most commonly used oral anticoagulant. Phenindione is an alternative, but is rarely used because of its potential for serious allergic reactions.

Warfarin acts by interfering with the formation of functionally normal coagulant factors II (prothrombin), VII, IX and X. The biological activity of these factors depends on the ability of vitamin K to convert glutamic acid residues to γ-carboxyglutamic acid residues. This confers on these coagulation factors the ability to bind calcium ions, allowing the proteins then to bind to phospholipids – an important prerequisite for the efficient function of the coagulation cascade. Warfarin blocks this vitamin K-dependent activity and prevents the formation of γ-carboxyglutamic acid residues. By a similar process, other vitamin K-dependent protein levels (e.g. proteins C and S) are also reduced in patients on warfarin.

Warfarin is completely absorbed from the small bowel and circulates loosely bound to albumin. It is degraded by enzymes on the hepatic endoplasmic reticulum, and these degraded products are excreted in the urine. No free warfarin appears in the urine. Warfarin crosses the placenta and appears in breast milk. The half-life of warfarin varies but has a mean value of 44 hours.

Anticoagulant control is monitored by the prothrombin time,

the results of which are given as the international normalized ratio (INR). This is designed to produce consistent and reproducible results in all laboratories, despite the use of different reagents. The recommended INR is 2–4.

High initial doses of warfarin are no longer recommended. With high drug doses, synthesis of factors II, VII, IX and X ceases, and they disappear from the blood according to their half-lives. Because the half-life of factor VII is only five hours, a very low factor VII level with a greatly prolonged INR will be observed. The levels of other coagulant factors will fall more slowly (half-life of factor II = 100 hours; half-life of factors IX and X = 20–30 hours). The initial rapid disappearance of factor VII may produce a bleeding tendency, but probably does not protect against thrombosis. In this regard, reduced levels of factors IX and X are more important, and that is why it takes three or four days to obtain a satisfactory anticoagulant effect from warfarin. A suitable regimen for starting warfarin is 10 mg daily for two days, followed by a smaller dose, e.g. 5 mg daily, adjusted depending on the INR. By this method, synthesis of coagulation factors is not completely suppressed, and a new equilibrium between synthesis and degradation is established.

The main side effect of warfarin is bleeding from renal, gastrointestinal and skin sites. Occasionally, retroperitoneal haemorrhage or subdural haematomas may occur. In those patients who bleed and whose INR is well controlled, an underlying cause should be sought. Bleeding may occur in those patients with a grossly prolonged INR. More frequently, patients will present with a prolonged INR but no clinical bleeding tendency, and in this situation it may be expedient simply to stop warfarin for a few days and restart again at a lower dosage regimen. In those patients who are bleeding, immediate correction of the INR can be achieved by an infusion of fresh frozen plasma. Warfarin effects may also be counteracted (and probably should be for any INR > 6) by intravenous vitamin K, but this may take 6–12 hours and it may render the patient intolerant to warfarin for 1–2 weeks afterwards. Other side effects of warfarin are rare and include gangrenous infarcts of the skin early in treatment and the purple toe syndrome, a bilateral painful discoloration of the toes. Both of these syndromes may be related to a reduction in protein C levels which occurs early after warfarin has been instituted and which may then, paradoxically, predispose a patient to thrombotic attacks.

Many drugs can interfere with the activity of warfarin. The British National Formulary should be consulted for further details of this. In addition, aspirin should be avoided because of its antiplatelet activity.

There may be difficulty in monitoring warfarin therapy in patients receiving heparin. As heparin may prolong the prothrombin time, problems may arise in determining the correct dose of warfarin for an individual patient. This problem only occurs when patients receive intravenous intermittent bolus doses of heparin. In this situation, a mid-day heparin dose should be omitted, and because of the short half-life of heparin, a prolonged prothrombin time measured eight hours after the last heparin dose can be regarded as due to warfarin effect. It is now more popular to use a continuous heparin infusion, and this will rarely produce a significant prolongation of the prothrombin time.

Pregnancy and Warfarin

A disadvantage of warfarin is that, unlike heparin, it crosses the placenta. This is associated with an increased risk of retroplacental and fetal intracerebral haemorrhage. In addition, it may cause chondrodysplasia punctata, fetal optic atrophy and microcephaly with mental retardation. In view of this, wafarin should probably not be used, especially in the first trimester of pregnancy, as heparin is a suitable and equally efficacious alternative except in patients with prosthetic heart valves.

Although warfarin is excreted in breast milk, it is present in such small quantities that the baby's coagulation profile is not altered, and therefore breast feeding in mothers taking warfarin is not contra-indicated.

HEPARIN

Heparin is usually the treatment of choice in the face of an acute clinical thrombotic attack because it acts immediately when given intravenously. The activity of heparin depends on the presence of antithrombin III (AT III), a naturally occurring anticoagulant. Heparin binds to AT III, producing conformational molecular changes and thereby greatly increasing the inhibitory action of AT III on thrombin and other activated coagulation factors.

Theoretically, heparin should not be effective in patients with very low AT III levels, but this is rarely a significant clinical problem. Conversely, AT III levels may fall during the first few days of treatment, although again, this is rarely a problem in practice.

Heparin can be given intravenously or subcutaneously. The intravenous route is preferred for initial therapy. Heparin can be given as intermittent bolus injections, but a continuous intravenous infusion (1000 U/hour) is to be preferred, because constant blood heparin levels are obtained. This may be associated with a lower incidence of significant bleeding episodes. The laboratory control of heparin is a controversial subject, and no firm advice can be given. Generally speaking, unlike the use of the INR in the control of warfarin therapy, no single laboratory test is universally used for the control of heparin therapy, but most laboratories use either the kaolin cephalin clotting time (KCCT) or thrombin time. Furthermore, there are no firm guidelines based on clinical trial material as to the circulating level of heparin to aim for. Perhaps this reflects the lack of correlation between the presence of bleeding episodes and coagulation results.

Subcutaneous or 'low-dose' heparin is used prophylactically in doses of 5000–10 000 U b.d. Injections are usually given into the anterior abdominal wall, and this form of treatment is used prophylactically during operative procedures or pregnancy.

The major side-effect of heparin is haemorrhage, which occurs in a small percentage of patients. Osteoporosis may occur in patients receiving long-term heparin. More recently, heparin-induced thrombocytopenia and arterial thrombosis have been described. With this complication, the initiating event appears to be an intravascular immune-mediated aggregation of platelets.

If bleeding occurs, stopping heparin (with its very short half-life of 60 minutes) is usually sufficient. Otherwise, circulating heparin can be neutralized by protamine sulphate (1 mg protamine neutralizes 1 mg [100 U] heparin). However, it is important to know that excess protamine acts as an anticoagulant, and allergic reactions are common.

More recently, heparins with a very low molecular weight have been introduced. These agents have maximum activity in inhibiting factor Xa and have less of a global inhibitory effect on the overall coagulation cascade compared with unfractionated heparin. It is hoped that these drugs will be as efficacious in treating and preventing thrombotic episodes as unfractionated heparin, but less harmful in terms of associated bleeding episodes. These matters are the subject of several trials at the present time.

ANCROD

This is a proteolytic enzyme which cleaves a specific small molecular weight fragment (fibrinopeptide A) from fibrinogen. Fibrin formed from this reaction is highly susceptible to fibrinolysis. Ancrod, therefore, produces a state of hypofibrinogenaemia and incoagulable blood. Following the breakdown of fibrin, fibrin degradation products rise initially and then fall to normal levels as circulating fibrinogen levels fall. This drug is given intravenously (1 U/kg over 12 hours followed by 0·5 U/kg every 12 hours). The effect of this drug can be monitored by measuring fibrinogen levels. A satisfactory fibrinogen level is about 0·5 g/l. Remarkably few side-effects are evident, and there is a lower incidence of bleeding complications when compared with either heparin or fibrinolytic drugs. Should bleeding occur, replacement therapy with fibrinogen is usually satisfactory. An antivenom is available but is rarely required.

FIBRINOLYTIC AGENTS

A major advantage of these drugs over other anticoagulants is their potential for removing intravascular fibrin clots and thus obtaining vascular patency. In this form of therapy, the fibrinolytic system is activated by an infusion of plasminogen activator, such as streptokinase or urokinase. However, these agents have not been as popular as the oral anticoagulants and heparin because of the difficulty in proving their superiority over these drugs and because of their high incidence of bleeding complications. The main indication for the use of fibrinolytic therapy has been massive pulmonary embolism, where the potential to achieve a rapid reversal of the vascular obstruction is required. In this situation, these drugs have proved superior to heparin in a number of trials. Recent evidence suggests that early fibrinolytic therapy reduces mortality after acute myocardial infarction.

Streptokinase is obtained from B-haemolytic streptococci. Its half-life is 30 minutes, and so it is rapidly cleared from the circulation. Antibodies to streptokinase are invariably present, presumably from previous streptococcal infections; a larger initial neutralizing dose must therefore be used. A recommended schedule is: 250 000 U intravenously, followed by 100 000 U/hour for 24 hours, followed by conventional anticoagulation. Urokinase has a half-life of 16 minutes when given as an infusion. However unlike streptokinase therapy, no universally accepted dose of urokinase has yet found favour.

The laboratory control of these agents is controversial. The thrombin time, which reflects hypofibrinogenaemia and raised fibrin degradation product levels, is probably the most suitable, and a four-fold prolongation of the thrombin time (compared with normal values) after the first six hours of treatment is considered satisfactory. Otherwise, maintaining plasma fibrinogen levels at about 0·5 g/l is adequate.

The major side effect of these drugs is bleeding, particularly at the site of catheter insertion. They must be avoided in patients with recent peptic ulceration or surgery. Avoidance of bleeding complications may be possible by reducing the number of invasive procedures during therapy and avoiding the use of other anticoagulant or antiplatelet agents. If significant bleeding occurs, because of the short half-life of these drugs all that is usually necessary is to stop the infusion. In rare situations, an antifibrinolytic agent such as tranexamic acid rapidly restores the situation to normal.

These problems may be overcome by the recent introduction of tissue plasminogen activator (TPA). This agent was originally produced from a human melanoma cell line but is now made available using DNA recombinant techniques. Like streptokinase and urokinase, it has a short half-life. However, unlike these drugs, which have an equal affinity for fibrin-bound or free plasminogen and thus produce a severe systemic haemostatic defect, TPA has a marked preference for fibrin-bound plasminogen and has a localized effect. TPA appears to be an effective coronary artery thrombolytic agent. A major advantage is that it is effective when given intravenously and does not need to be delivered directly into the coronary circulation. The incidence of haemorrhage appears to be very low when compared with streptokinase and urokinase, and although it may produce a moderate reduction in fibrinogen and other coagulation factor levels, these changes are not clinically significant.

ANTIPLATELET DRUGS

The use of these drugs is based on the recognition that platelets have a role to play in the development of thrombotic disease, especially that arising in the arterial vascular tree. A number of drugs interfere with platelet function as demonstrated in the laboratory, but to assess their effectiveness in clinical trials has, in many situations, been difficult and inconclusive.

Aspirin

This drug acts by inhibiting cyclo-oxygenase activity and thereby reduces prostaglandin synthesis in platelets. While marked changes in platelet aggregation in vitro can be demonstrated, changes in platelet survival in vivo have not been shown. A single dose of aspirin irreversibly affects platelets and megakaryocytes, and therefore the return of normal platelet function will depend on the formation of a new, unaffected cohort of platelets, which usually takes 5-7 days. Normal doses of aspirin not only affect platelets but also reduce prostacyclin formation within vascular endothelial cells. Prostacyclin is an agent capable of inhibiting platelet aggregation – hence the use of 'mini' doses of aspirin (75 mg daily or on alternate days) in an attempt to spare vascular endothelial cells from its effect. Whether this is so, and whether there is any clinical benefit from such an approach, remains to be seen.

Dipyridamole

Dipyridamole reduces platelet phosphodiesterase activity and raises intraplatelet cyclic AMP levels. It has a beneficial effect on platelet survival and has been assessed in many trials, frequently in addition to aspirin. There is little evidence to suggest that this drug has a significant antithrombotic effect.

Sulphinpyrazone

The mechanism of action of this agent is unclear, but it is thought to work through an effect on prostaglandin synthesis. It affects in vitro platelet function and also appears to correct in vivo platelet survival.

Ticlopidine

Ticlopidine has a beneficial effect on platelet survival and also alters in vitro platelet function. These effects are seen 1–2 days after drug administration and may persist for several days after the drug has been discontinued.

Prostacyclin

Prostacyclin and prostacyclin analogues are currently under investigation as antithrombotic agents because of their powerful adverse influence on platelet function.

These antiplatelet drugs have now been evaluated in most forms of arterial and venous thrombotic disease. The majority of the studies have been inconclusive or have been criticized on methodological and/or statistical grounds. The following statements can be made, however:

1. Aspirin is highly effective in reversing digital ischaemia which occasionally complicates essential thrombocythaemia.
2. Warfarin and dipyridamole are of use in patients who have received prosthetic heart valves.
3. Aspirin may be effective in patients with transient ischaemic attacks (TIA), reducing not only the number of such attacks but also the incidence of cerebrovascular accidents and death in those patients. There appears to be a sex preference, males benefiting more than females from aspirin treatment for TIA.
4. Sulphinpyrazone may help to prevent arteriovenous shunt thrombosis.
5. Antiplatelet agents may help to prevent post-aortocoronary bypass graft thrombosis.
6. It is debatable whether aspirin or sulphinpyrazone are effective in preventing coronary artery thrombosis.

7. Surprisingly, aspirin may have some efficacy in preventing venous thrombosis in the postoperative situation. At the present time, such an approach must be considered as experimental and could not be generally recommended.

FURTHER READING

Kelton K.G. (1983). Antiplatelet agents: rationale and results. *Clinics in Haematology*, **12**(1), 311–345.

Letsky E.A. (1975). Thromboembolism in pregnancy and its management. *Br. J. Haematol.* **57**, 543–550.

Prentice C.R.M. (1975). Indications for antifibrinolytic therapy. *Thrombos. Diathes. Haemorrh.*, **34**, 634–641.

Wessler S., Gitel S.N. (1984). Warfarin. From bedside to bench. *New Engl. J. Med.*, **311**, 645–652.

Chapter Twenty Five

Liver Disease and Haematology

INTRODUCTION

In the embryo, the liver is an important site of blood formation, but this function is lost before birth. However, the liver continues throughout life to be the site of synthesis of many coagulation factors, and also a major site of removal of activated coagulation factors, fibrinolytic enzymes and fibrin degradation products. Thrombocytopenia is commonly present in association with liver disease and, in combination with coagulation disorders, may lead to generalized bleeding problems. Recognition of changes in the blood indices and blood film are important, as they may give the first hint of liver disease.

HEPATITIS

Virus hepatitis may be accompanied in the first few days of clinical illness with a reactive neutrophilia, which is usually replaced within a week by a reactive lymphocytosis. Glandular fever complicated by hepatitis usually causes lymphocytosis with atypical mononuclear cells, but a similar appearance is occasionally seen with hepatitis caused by other viruses, which can be distinguished by antibody studies.

At the height of the illness, a mild haemolytic anaemia may occur and a slight transient thrombocytopenia is common, as with any virus infection.

A rare but important complication of hepatitis is aplastic anaemia, which presents with falling haemoglobin levels (with low reticulocyte counts) in the weeks after the initial illness, followed by falling neutrophil and platelet counts. The aplasia produced is usually profound and carries an extremely poor prognosis (over 80 per cent die within one year). Where a donor is available, bone marrow transplantation should not be delayed, as the results are best if treatment is instituted before the patient has received multiple transfusions and has become generally ill.

CHRONIC ACTIVE HEPATITIS

In this chronic inflammatory disorder, a mild anaemia with raised plasma viscosity is found. On occasions, the disease is complicated by an auto-immune haemolytic anaemia characterized by the appearance of spherocytes, a positive Coombs' test and an antibody active at blood temperature. A mild pancytopenia sometimes occurs, which may reflect hypersplenism.

OBSTRUCTIVE JAUNDICE

Chronic obstruction from any cause may alter plasma lipids. These interchange freely with the red cell membrane surface, increasing its cholesterol and lecithin content. The resulting increase in the area of the surface of the cell results in the appearance of large numbers of target cells in the blood film. Cross-transfusion studies show that the changes in the red cell are acquired in the circulation (and may be lost rapidly if the cells are transfused into a normal person).

PORTAL HYPERTENSION

Splenomegaly, with its sequestration and destruction of blood elements, causes mild anaemia and neutropenia, which are usually of no great clinical importance. Red cell pooling may add to the anaemia. Thrombocytopenia aggravates the coagulation problems caused by underlying liver disease, and bleeding may be serious, particularly if there are oesophageal varices.

CHRONIC LIVER FAILURE AND CIRRHOSIS

The first suspicion of cirrhosis may be aroused by an abnormal blood film, leucopenia, thrombocytopenia or a prolonged prothrombin time.

Anaemia has many causes, often present in combination (*see* Table 25.1). It is frequently microcytic due to iron deficiency, reflecting a poor diet, or bleeding problems. By contrast, a macrocytic picture is also common and reflects liver dysfunction, alcohol ingestion or folate deficiency. Mild degrees of liver impairment, particularly if there is an obstructive element, cause anaemia with target cells, produced by increased red cell membrane phospholipids and cholesterol. This may be associated with a moderate increase in red cell size (up to 115 fl). More severe liver failure produces a very different blood picture of a haemolytic anaemia associated with very irregular spiky red cells (acanthocytes or spur cells), with an increased cholesterol to phospholipid ratio. These rigid cells are lysed prematurely in the spleen or even in the circulation, with resultant haemoglobinuria and haemosiderinuria. Spur cell anaemia is associated with a very poor prognosis. Splenic pooling and hypersplenism may contribute to the other causes of anaemia.

Thrombocytopenia and leucopenia are usually a result of hypersplenism, but deficiency of folic acid should not be overlooked.

Coagulation disorders are considered below.

Table 25.1
ANAEMIA WITH CIRRHOSIS AND LIVER FAILURE

Microcytic	Iron deficiency (mainly from bleeding)
Macrocytic	Alcohol, folate deficiency

Normocytic	Target cell (especially obstructive; may be macrocytic)
	Splenic pooling
	Haemolytic
	  Hypersplenism
	  Spur cell anaemia (severe liver failure)
	  Zieve's syndrome (acute alcohol abuse)

Dimorphic	Sideroblastic (alcohol)

HAEMATOLOGICAL EFFECTS OF ALCOHOL

Macrocytosis is a very common finding in alcohol abuse and may be the only abnormality to suggest the problem. The macrocytosis is typically round and uniform (in vitamin B_{12} or folate deficiency the macrocytes are typically oval with marked anisocytosis, and the neutrophils are hypersegmented). The macrocytosis can develop after only a few days of heavy drinking and may last for some weeks even in non-alcoholics with no underlying liver disorder; the mean corpuscular volume (MCV) is therefore useful in following the success of attempts to reduce the alcohol intake. As chronic alcoholics often have a poor diet, folate deficiency may complicate the direct toxic effects of alcohol.

Zieve described a syndrome of acute alcoholic abuse followed by a haemolytic anaemia with frequent target cells, raised reticulocytes, raised bilirubin and raised plasma triglyceride and cholesterol levels. The liver shows fatty change, and the syndrome resolves over a few days.

In some severe alcoholics, a sideroblastic marrow is found, presenting either as a dysplastic macrocytic anaemia or with a dimorphic blood picture showing dysplastic microcytes and macrocytes in the blood film. These toxic changes disappear on withdrawal.

It is thought that alcohol can directly cause neutropenia and thrombocytopenia, but it is usually difficult to assess the relative contribution of alcohol, folate deficiency and hypersplenism.

DISORDERS OF COAGULATION

Coagulation disorders (Table 25.2) may increase bleeding from known gastro-intestinal lesions or, if severe, can cause spontaneous bleeding into the skin and mucosal surfaces. Laboratory tests reveal some coagulation disorder in most patients with liver disease, but clinical bleeding problems are found in only about 15 per cent of these patients. The detailed nature of the coagulation problem is usually complex, but simple tests can give helpful guides to treatment and prognosis.

Thrombocytopenia, except when due to massive transfusion, suggests hypersplenism, folate deficiency, alcohol abuse or disseminated intravascular coagulation (DIC). A platelet count below about $50 \times 10^9/l$ may contribute to bleeding problems

Table 25.2
BLEEDING AND LIVER DISEASE

Hypersplenism	Thrombocytopenia (other factors may contribute)
Obstructive jaundice	Vitamin K deficiency leading to low factors II, VII, IX and X (corrected by vitamin K)
Hepatocellular disease	Cell damage leading to low factors II, VII, IX and X (only partially corrected by vitamin K) and if severe, to low factors I, V and XIII Dysfibrinogenaemia
Miscellaneous	Disseminated intravascular coagulation

(particularly if coagulation problems are also present), and platelet infusions may help.

In obstructive jaundice, vitamin K is poorly absorbed because of the absence of bile salts, and the vitamin K-dependent coagulation factors (II, VII, IX and X) fall, resulting in bleeding problems if levels below about 10 per cent of normal are found. The prothrombin time (which is raised with deficient levels of factors I, II, V, VII and X) is a sensitive index of this problem, which can be completely reversed by parenteral vitamin K administration (e.g. phytomenadione 10 mg/day intramuscularly for three days) if liver cell function is good.

Vitamin K is needed for the carboxylation of glutamic acid in the precursor molecules of the appropriate factors. In vitamin K deficiency (and during oral anticoagulant therapy), abnormal proteins called PIVKA (protein induced by vitamin K absence) are produced, which cause a rather excessive prolongation of the Thrombotest time. The prothrombin time is therefore clearly preferable in this situation as a measure of vitamin K-dependent factors.

In hepatocellular disease, these same factors are decreased, and the prothrombin time has proved to be a useful indicator of the extent of liver damage; it also has prognostic significance (e.g. in cirrhosis, hepatic coma, hepatitis and paracetamol poisoning).

The obstructive element can again be corrected by vitamin K, but some abnormality, reflecting liver cell necrosis, often remains. A slight prolongation of the prothrombin time (e.g. by three seconds) is usually taken as a contra-indication to liver biopsy, unless it can be corrected. If this is not achieved by vitamin K administration (which takes over six hours to act), fresh frozen plasma is sometime used and acts immediately, but for only a few hours because of the short half-life of factor VII (five hours). Where plasma volume is a problem, prothrombin complex concentrates have been infused, but unfortunately, these may contain activated factors which can trigger DIC and thromboembolism.

In severe liver damage, factors I, V and XIII, which are also synthesized in the liver, may also be reduced and can be treated by infusions, but usually with little clinical improvement.

In about 50 per cent of patients with moderate hepatocellular disease, an abnormal fibrinogen with excess sialic acid is synthesized, which gives normal immunological levels of fibrinogen but a prolonged thrombin or reptilase time.

Although there is a large literature on disseminated intravascular lysis and fibrinolysis in liver disease, the results of investigation for these states, which are often present in some degree, seldom lead to any advantage in therapy.

FURTHER READING

Brunt P.W., Losowsky M.S., Read A.E. (1984). *The Liver and Biliary System.* London: Heinemann Medical Books.

Chapter Twenty Six

Renal Disease and Haematology

A variety of haematological complications may accompany renal disease.

ANAEMIA

Severe anaemia (6–7 g/dl) is characteristically seen in patients with chronic renal failure. The degree of anaemia is not directly related to the degree of uraemia, but a rough parallel exists. The anaemia is usually of a normochromic, normocytic type accompanied by low numbers of reticulocytes. The morphology of the red cells is usually unremarkable, but occasionally spiculated cells (Burr cells) may be seen. Patients can tolerate very low haemoglobin levels remarkably well, perhaps because of an accompanying increased intracellular concentration of 2,3-diphosphoglycerate, which decreases the affinity of haemoglobin for oxygen. Therefore, there is no impairment in the ability of red cells to act as oxygen carriers.

The cause of this anaemia is multifactorial. Factors such as a reduced red cell survival, blood loss associated with dialysis, iron and folate deficiency and, possibly, aluminium toxicity contribute, but the main problem is an absence of an appropriate increase in erythropoietin production in response to anaemia. This is not surprising, as the main site of erythropoietin production is the kidney.

Treatment of severe anaemia in chronic renal failure has up to now been unsatisfactory. Blood transfusions have been avoided where possible because of the problems of fluid and iron overload and hepatitis transmission. Iron is given when a deficiency has been identified, and folic acid is given routinely, especially in those patients undergoing dialysis. Androgens may be helpful in raising haemoglobin levels, but have not gained general acceptance because of side effects, such as oedema, hirsutism and cholestasis.

A major advance has been the production of erythropoietin by recombinant DNA technology. Early studies have shown that this agent can correct the anaemia of chronic renal failure, and it appears to be associated with few, if any, side effects. It may also improve the haemostatic defect in these patients, but whether erythropoietin, by correcting the anaemia, increases the risk of thrombotic events remains to be seen.

HAEMOSTATIC DEFECTS

A severe bleeding disorder may occur in patients with untreated renal failure. Although modest abnormalities in coagulation factor profiles and thrombocytopenia may occasionally be present, it is now generally accepted that the major cause of bleeding is a qualitative platelet defect. This defect does not closely correlate with the degree of uraemia or the type of underlying renal disease present.

A variety of platelet functional defects have been described. These include a prolonged bleeding time, a failure of platelets to develop normal procoagulant activity after suitable stimuli, an impairment of platelet adherence to foreign surfaces and abnormal aggregation responses to a variety of aggregating agents.

The precise cause of this platelet defect is unknown. It has been proposed that increased plasma levels of either guanidosuccinic acid, phenols or urea are responsible, but there is no agreement on this. More recently, a lack of factor VIII or a lack of large molecular weight molecules of factor VIII von Willebrand factor has been suggested, particularly in view of the therapeutic response to cryoprecipitate and deamino-8-D-arginine vasopressin (DDAVP). However, this has not been demonstrated to date.

It is generally accepted that the best indicator of those patients who are likely to be bleeders is a prolonged bleeding time. Most patients have abnormal in vitro aggregation responses, and this has not been a helpful discriminatory factor. Fortunately, dialysis predictably corrects the haemostatic defect in most patients, and platelet function returns to normal 24–48 hours after. Although the reason is unclear, both cryoprecipitate and DDAVP have been shown to produce a significant but transient reduction in the bleeding time in some patients, allowing surgery to be performed without the occurrence of excessive bleeding. Conjugated oestrogens have a similar effect, with a more prolonged duration of action.

POLYCYTHAEMIA

Polycythaemia is a not infrequent complication of hypernephroma, renal cysts (either solitary or polycystic renal disease or hydronephrosis), renal artery stenosis and transplant rejections. Clinically, this presents as an erythrocytosis with normal white blood cell and platelet counts. Hepatosplenomegaly is not present, and a marrow biopsy should not demonstrate any increase in reticulin. A red cell mass and plasma volume estimation will demonstrate the presence of true polycythaemia. The cause in most cases is likely to be an increased production of erythropoietin from the involved kidney, and correction of the polycythaemia usually accompanies successful treatment of the underlying disease.

THROMBOTIC THROMBOCYTOPENIC PURPURA AND HAEMOLYTIC URAEMIC SYNDROME

Thrombotic thrombocytopenic purpura (TTP) is a disease of adults and is characterized by fever, progressive renal failure, neurological abnormalities, haemolytic anaemia and thrombocytopenia. Haemolytic uraemic syndrome (HUS) is normally a disease of children and is characterized by renal failure, thrombocytopenia and haemolytic anaemia. It is frequently preceded by a febrile illness. In both diseases, the thrombocytopenia is of a consumptive type, and the haemolysis is of a micro-angiopathic type, characteristically with many fragmented red cells on the blood film.

TTP is a heterogeneous syndrome and can be found in association with systemic lupus erythematosus, the contraceptive pill, pregnancy and cyclosporin A therapy.

While there are clinical differences between these two diseases (e.g. neurological abnormalities in TTP, and a predilection for renal involvement with frequent sparing of other tissues in HUS), it is generally thought that the underlying pathophysiology is similar, the main event being the deposition of platelet/fibrin thrombi in the microcirculation with resultant tissue damage. It has been postulated that this may follow primary damage to vascular endothelial cells. Recently, reduced prostacyclin synthesis/release from endothelial cells has been suggested as a possible cause for intravascular platelet deposition. A deficiency of a plasma stimulating substance, necessary for the optimal production and release of prostacyclin from endothelial cells, has been demonstrated in TTP patients.

Without treatment, the mortality rate is very high in severe cases. The primary form of treatment relates to plasma manipulation and a 60–70 per cent response rate follows a daily infusion of 6–8 units of fresh frozen plasma. A response is usually seen within 48–72 hours. Relapses may occur following the discontinuation of treatment, and an occasional patient requires maintenance fresh frozen plasma infusions. If no response to plasma infusions occurs within 48 hours, then plasma exchange with fresh frozen plasma replacement gives a 60–80 per cent response rate. Should both of these measures fail, prostacyclin infusions have been tried (because of the reduced release of prostacyclin from endothelial cells), although with mixed success.

RENAL DISEASE IN MULTIPLE MYELOMA

The kidney is frequently affected in this disease. Raised blood urea and creatinine levels at presentation, which are not normalized by rehydration, are a bad prognostic sign. Patients who present with acute oliguric renal failure, do particularly badly, although anecdotal reports of improvement following dialysis and chemotherapy have occurred.

Frequently, patients present with mild to moderate renal failure. This is associated with excessive quantities of free monoclonal light chains (i.e. Bence–Jones protein) being excreted through the kidneys. They are reabsorbed by the renal tubules and cause toxic damage to these structures. Other causes of renal disease include hypercalcaemia, hyperuricaemia, amyloid deposition and infection. Dehydration may rapidly exacerbate pre-existing renal failure, and immobilization should be avoided, as this may precipitate hypercalcaemia in these patients.

A recent Medical Research Council study has demonstrated the importance of prolonged fluid replacement therapy (three litres daily at least) on renal function in this disease. Otherwise, chemotherapy and the avoidance of the other precipitating factors mentioned above should stabilize and control the degree of renal failure, at least for a while.

RENAL TRANSPLANTATION

Thrombocytopenia with a micro-angiopathic haemolytic anaemia has been reported as a likely predictor of rejection. Cyclosporin may produce a TTP-like syndrome. Azathioprine, an inhibitor of purine synthesis, may produce anaemia, leucopenia or thrombocytopenia. It can produce marked bone marrow megaloblastic changes not related to either vitamin B_{12} or folic acid deficiency.

Polyclonal hyperplasia of lymphoid tissues, perhaps related to Epstein–Barr virus infection, and lymphomas occur with increased frequency after renal transplantation. The lymphomas typically are derived from B-lymphocytes, are of a high grade malignant type and occur in unusual anatomical sites, such as the central nervous system. They are frequently resistant to therapy.

SICKLE-CELL DISEASE AND SICKLE TRAIT

The environment of the renal medulla, i.e. stasis, hyperosmolality, low pH and hypoxia, is particularly well suited to produce sickling of red cells. In sickle trait, a remarkably benign condition, the kidney is the only organ affected. Many patients show reduced urine concentrating ability and recurrent haematuria, presumably secondary to small infarctions. In the more serious sickle-cell disease, renal infarcts, renal papillary necrosis and recurrent urinary tract infections are common. The natural history of renal disease in sickle-cell disease is unknown, and it remains to be seen if renal failure will eventually occur in these patients. Unfortunately, there is no treatment available which prevents the occurrence of the sickling phenomenon.

FURTHER READING

Carvalho A.C. (1983). Bleeding in uraemia – a clinical challenge. *New Engl. J. Med.*, **308**, 38–39.

Machin S.J. (1984). Thrombotic thrombocytopenic purpura. *Br. J. Haematol.*, **56**, 191–195.

Chapter Twenty Seven

Topics in Paediatric Haematology

A detailed discussion of blood disorders in children is outside the scope of this chapter. However, an attempt is made to stress the important differences in normal haematological values between children and adults and to select a number of topics of particular interest or importance.

'PHYSIOLOGICAL' CHANGES IN THE BLOOD COUNT DURING CHILDHOOD

Compared with the adult, the normal full-term neonate is polycythaemic and macrocytic (mean haemoglobin 18·4 g/dl and mean corpuscular volume (MCV) 108 fl on the first day of life). The higher red cell count reflects adaptation to the relatively hypoxic intra-uterine environment and the predominance of high oxygen affinity fetal haemoglobin (haemoglobin F). During the first weeks of life, there is a gradual fall in haemoglobin concentration to a nadir of 8·0 to 10·0 g/dl at 8–12 weeks of age. This 'physiological anaemia of infancy' is accompanied by reticulocytopenia and grossly reduced erythroid activity in the marrow. Treatment with iron or other haematinics produces no rise in haemoglobin. Current evidence suggests that, after delivery, the oxygen carrying capacity of the infant's blood at ambient oxygen tension is vastly in excess of requirements and that the erythropoietin drive to red cell production is 'switched off'. When the haemoglobin concentration (abetted by the progressive switch to lower oxygen affinity adult haemoglobin A) falls to the appropriate level, erythropoiesis is resumed. Despite this impressive fall in haemoglobin, data suggest that the capacity for oxygen transport rises from the moment of birth. Infants born prematurely show a more marked fall in haemoglobin and reach the nadir earlier (at 6–8 weeks after delivery). Although controversial, recent evidence suggests that premature infants have impaired regulation of erythropoietin and that the haemoglobin may fall to distinctly 'unphysiological' levels, which merit treatment by transfusion.

In addition to macrocytosis, the red cells of the normal neonate show marked anisocytosis and poikilocytosis with frequent target cells, acanthocytes and spherocytes. Nucleated red cells are present in small numbers but normally disappear from the peripheral circulation in the first four or five days of life. These morphological changes reflect a combination of immature red cell enzyme systems (with reduced erythrocyte life-span) and low functional capacity of the spleen and reticulo-endothelial system (impaired 'quality control')

In the first three days of life, the mean white cell count is $20 \times 10^9/l$, with 50–70 per cent granulocytes and occasional metamyelocytes and myelocytes. In the first four years of life, the total white cell count is close to normal adult level, but lymphocytes comprise 50–60 per cent of the leucocytes. The normal adult differential count is reached between four and six years of age. Serious bacterial infection in the neonate is often not accompanied by the neutrophilia characteristic of adults and older children. However, an increase in the proportion of immature 'band' neutrophils may be of great value in differential diagnosis. Severe leucopenia in the presence of serious bacterial infection is a very poor prognostic indicator in the neonate. Pronounced lymphocytosis in the older child is a feature of many virus infections, particularly infectious mononucleosis, cytomegalovirus, toxoplasmosis and pertussis.

The platelet count in infancy and childhood is similar to normal adult values ($150–400 \times 10^9/l$).

NEONATAL THROMBOCYTOPENIA

Neonatal thrombocytopenia is common in hospital practice (Table 27.1). It is most often seen in the sick premature neonate with infection, respiratory distress syndrome or birth asphyxia in whom there may be evidence of disseminated intravascular coagulation (DIC). Thrombocytopenia is a frequent accompaniment of congenital (maternally derived) infection, the most

Table 27.1
CAUSES OF NEONATAL THROMBOCYTOPENIA

Secondary to infection
   Bacterial (may be associated with DIC)
   Congenital (TORCH complex, syphilis)

Immune
   Auto-immune
   Iso-immune (usually anti-Pl^{A1})

Inherited platelet disorder
   Bernard–Soulier syndrome
   May–Hegglin syndrome
   Wiskott–Aldrich syndrome
   Thrombocytopenia—absent radius (TAR) syndrome

Miscellaneous
   DIC (infection, shock, asphyxia etc.)
   Maternal drugs (e.g. alcohol, thiazide diuretics)
   Post-exchange transfusion
   Marrow infiltration by malignant disease (rare)
   Phototherapy
   Indwelling catheter

DIC = disseminated intravascular coagulation; TORCH = toxoplasmosis, rubella, cytomegalovirus, herpes simplex.

common causes in British practice being toxoplasmosis, rubella, cytomegalovirus and herpes simplex (the TORCH complex), although congenital syphilis must not be forgotten.

Auto-immune thrombocytopenia is seen in the infants of mothers with idiopathic thrombocytopenic purpura or diseases such as systemic lupus erythematosus in which maternal IgG auto-antibodies may cross the placenta (*see* Chapter 28). Two important clinical points are that a normal maternal platelet count does not rule out the presence of significant antibodies, especially if splenectomy has been performed, and that the infant's platelet count may fall steeply in the first 48 hours of life. High-dose intravenous immunoglobulin (IVIG) therapy of the mother in late pregnancy may be the treatment of choice for maximum protection of mother and infant (Chapter 28). Iso-immune thrombocytopenia is usually seen in the infants of the two per cent of women who lack the platelet-specific Pl^{A1} antigen. The mother is sensitized by fetomaternal haemorrhage containing Pl^{A1}-positive platelets (analogous to haemolytic disease of the newborn), and 'immune' IgG antibodies cross the placenta and affect the infant. A serious bleeding disorder is seen in the infant, with reported mortality rates of up to 15 per cent from cerebral haemorrhage. As with auto-immune thrombocytopenia, the process is essentially self-limiting, as maternal antibody levels in the infant decay over the first two to six weeks of life. Iso-immune thrombocytopenia may occur in the first pregnancy and is clearly unpredictable in this instance. However, after an initial affected pregnancy, it can be assumed that all subsequent pregnancies will be at risk (particularly if the father is homozygous for the Pl^{A1} antigen). Once again, the use of IVIG administered to the mother in late, or even throughout, pregnancy may be effective in preventing severe fetal and maternal thrombocytopenia. Administration of IVIG to the infant is often effective and may replace the less convenient and more hazardous treatment of exchange transfusion and transfusion of washed maternal platelets.

Phototherapy may cause a fall in neonatal platelet count (direct toxicity), and maternal drug ingestion (e.g. thiazides, penicillins) may affect the infant.

Inherited thrombocytopenias are rare. Distinctive syndromes with qualitative platelet abnormalities may be recognized, such as the Bernard–Soulier and May–Hegglin syndromes (large platelets) or the Wiskott–Aldrich syndrome (small platelets). In the autosomal recessive thrombocytopenia–absent radius (TAR) syndrome, the thrombocytopenia is accompanied by bilateral hypoplasia of the radius; dislocated hips are common, and marrow megakaryocytes are reduced in number.

IDIOPATHIC THROMBOCYTOPENIC PURPURA IN CHILDHOOD

Compared with the adult form of this syndrome, childhood idiopathic thrombocytopenic purpura (ITP) more often follows an acute febrile (presumably viral) illness and generally pursues a benign self-limiting course. Presentation is often with sudden onset of widespread purpura and ecchymoses, and it is not uncommon for the suspicion of non-accidental injury to be raised. The most feared complication of childhood ITP is intracerebral haemorrhage, although many large series have shown the risk to be very small. The majority of children with mild purpura clearly require no treatment, and the platelet count recovers within a few weeks of onset. By six months after presentation, more than 90 per cent have shown complete resolution of the disease, and relapse is uncommon. Despite the overwhelmingly benign prognosis, it is difficult to avoid offering treatment to the child with 'wet' purpura, mucous membrane bleeding and a platelet count less than $20 \times 10^9/1$, although there is no controlled trial evidence to suggest benefit. In this situation, it is common practice to give steroids in the form of oral prednisolone 0·5–1·0 mg/kg, tailing off over 2–4 weeks. Steroids produce a rise in platelets in most cases, although levels may fall back as the dose is reduced. Hazardous, long-term administration of steroids should be avoided in this essentially benign disorder. There has been recent enthusiasm for the administration of high-dose IVIG to children presenting with ITP. IVIG produces a rapid, but usually temporary, improvement in the platelet count, and some authors claim a higher incidence of permanent remission. However, IVIG is very expensive, and the long-term immunological and microbiological consequences of treatment are unknown. Splenectomy is rarely indicated in childhood ITP, and less than five per cent of children will prove to have the adult form of chronic relapsing disease. Although the diagnosis of ITP may be made on the basis of clinical features and isolated thrombocytopenia on the blood film, it is the present author's view that bone marrow aspiration should be carried out in all cases where steroid therapy is contemplated. The major purpose of bone marrow examination in childhood ITP is to exclude the presence of acute lymphoblastic leukaemia, which may rarely present with thrombocytopenia alone. Such cases may respond temporarily to steroids, but this suboptimal treatment will prejudice the chances of long-term cure. The presence of a normal marrow is also highly reassuring to both the physician and parents, especially when a policy of non-intervention is pursued.

HAEMOLYTIC DISEASE OF THE NEWBORN

Maternal red cell allo-antibodies of the IgG class may cross the placenta and cause haemolytic anaemia in the fetus. The mother is sensitized to antigens absent from her own red cells by one of several mechanisms. Fetal red cells may enter the maternal circulation at the time of delivery or during the course of pregnancy. Obstetric manoeuvres, such as external version, amniocentesis and termination of pregnancy, may cause transplacental haemorrhage. Transfusion of incompatible blood or blood products may also result in allo-immunization. The most common antibodies causing haemolytic disease of the newborn (HDNB) are in the rhesus or ABO systems, but rarer cases in many other groups are described. The rate of haemolysis declines after delivery of the infant, as maternally derived antibody levels fall.

Rhesus Haemolytic Diseases of the Newborn

Rhesus (Rh) HDNB is due to the sensitization of Rh-D-negative mothers to the Rh(D) antigen in previous pregnancy or after incompatible blood transfusion. First pregnancies are rarely affected, and the clinical problem is usually due to a secondary immune response with rising anti-D antibody titres. Only 15 per cent of the native UK population lack the D-antigen, and the incidence of Rh-incompatible matings is approximately 12·5 per cent. However, even before routine prophylaxis against sensitization was available, the incidence of severely affected pregnancies was only 0·5 to 0·75 per cent (although this was a very significant cause of fetal wastage). The discrepancy in incidence relates to the apparent protective effect of coexisting ABO incompatibility, i.e. Rh-positive cells are removed more rapidly from the maternal circulation and may not produce sensitization, and only about 20 per cent of women are capable of producing high titre, biologically active anti-D antibodies in response to allo-immunization. The clinical severity of rhesus HDNB is highly variable (Table 27.2). At its most severe, there is fetal death in utero due to severe anaemia and hydrops foetalis. The liveborn infant may develop progressive jaundice during the first 24 hours of life, with the risk of severe neurological damage (kernicterus) if the level of unconjugated bilirubin exceeds the binding capacity of serum albumin and is deposited in the central nervous system. The classical blood film appearance in rhesus HDNB is 'erythroblastosis foetalis', with large numbers of nucleated red blood cells and a reticulocyte count up to 40 per cent. The direct antiglobulin (Coombs') test is usually positive in cord blood, indicating the presence of antibody on the infant's red cells.

Table 27.2
THE OUTCOME OF UNTREATED RHESUS HAEMOLYTIC DISEASE OF THE NEWBORN

50 %	– mildly affected; minimal haemolysis despite positive direct antiglobulin test.
25 %	– moderately affected; anaemia and hyperbilirubinaemia in the first days of life. Exchange transfusion may be needed.
25 %	– severely affected; fetuses die of hydrops foetalis (50 % before the 32nd week of gestation).

Routine antenatal tests should include checking the maternal rhesus group and screening for the presence of anti-D and any other 'irregular' antibodies. Rhesus(D)-negative women are monitored at least twice during pregnancy for the development of anti-D antibodies. Those with antibodies present, or with a past history of affected infants, are monitored closely for evidence of a rising titre. Precise indications for medical intervention during the pregnancy are controversial and vary with the expertise available at individual centres (Table 27.3). The risk of a severely affected fetus appears to be low if maternal anti-D levels remain below 4 iu/ml. The increasing ability of neonatal units to support infants of low gestational age has made a major contribution to the prognosis of pregnancies affected by rhesus HDNB. Efforts are directed to maintaining a viable fetus until it can be delivered at the earliest safe opportunity. The timing of delivery depends on a comparison of the relative risks of continued exposure to maternal antibody in utero and the probability of survival after premature delivery of the infant. An indication of the degree of haemolysis in the fetus can be obtained by measuring the optical density of amniotic fluid collected by amniocentesis. Standard nomograms derived by Liley are used to determine whether the

Table 27.3
THERAPEUTIC OPTIONS IN RHESUS HAEMOLYTIC DISEASE OF THE NEWBORN

Intra-uterine transfusion (via fetoscopy or peritoneal)
Early delivery and support
Plasma exchange
Exchange transfusion (postnatal)

fetus is in high, medium or low risk categories. Severely affected pregnancies may be sustained by intra-uterine transfusion of the fetus with Rh(D)-negative red cells. As peritoneal infusion of red cells can rarely be performed before the 26th week of pregnancy, amniocentesis is usually not indicated before this time. Amniocentesis itself carries a risk of precipitating fetomaternal haemorrhage and stimulating antibody production, and intra-uterine transfusion carries a not inconsiderable mortality, especially in less experienced hands. Patients with very high anti-D titres or a history of previous severely affected pregnancies may be helped by intensive plasma exchange throughout pregnancy, although the value of this treatment remains controversial. Dangerous degrees of hyperbilirubinaemia in the neonate are usually treated by exchange transfusion, using Rh(D)-negative red cells compatible in cross-match with the maternal serum. The purpose of exchange transfusion is to remove antibody-coated red cells and free plasma antibodies, to correct anaemia and to reduce bilirubin.

Clearly, prevention of rhesus HDNB is greatly preferable to attempts at dealing with the consequences of the disease. The introduction of prophylactic administration of Rh anti-D immunoglobulin postnatally to all rhesus-negative mothers has produced a dramatic fall in the incidence of this disorder. Anti-D immunoglobulin is given intramuscularly within 72 hours of delivery. The rapid removal of fetal D-positive cells from the maternal circulation before immunization occurs may be its major activity. A standard dose of 500 iu will cover a transplacental haemorrhage of up to 4 ml of fetal cells. A Kleihauer test is carried out on the mother's blood to determine the approximate volume of fetomaternal haemorrhage and thus allow the administration of larger amounts of anti-D immunoglobulin where necessary (125 iu will eliminate approximately 1 ml of red cells). Anti-D, usually in a dose of 50–250 iu, should be given after any potentially sensitizing obstetric manoeuvre, including termination of pregnancy, in rhesus-negative mothers. The most common cause of failure of anti-D prophylaxis in current practice is administrative failure to ensure that the immunoglobulin was given appropriately. Where postnatal anti-D immunoglobulin is given correctly, the failure rate is approximately 0·7 per cent per pregnancy. This failure rate can be further reduced by giving anti-D antenatally, for example at 28 and 34 weeks of pregnancy. The latter approach may be of a special benefit in primiparae where the sensitization rate can be brought down to the order of 0·16 per cent. There are no adverse effects on the fetus of administering anti-D antenatally.

ABO Haemolytic Disease of the Newborn

In approximately 15 per cent of pregnancies, the mother is blood group O and the fetus group A or B. However, clinically significant haemolytic disease is uncommon for several reasons: most naturally occurring anti-A or anti-B antibodies are IgM and cannot cross the placenta; only about 20 per cent of group O individuals will readily produce IgG antibodies which may affect the fetus; and A and B antigens are only poorly developed on fetal and neonatal red cells. Mild jaundice and anaemia due to ABO incompatibility is seen in about one in 25 of at-risk pregnancies, although the direct antiglobulin test is positive in up to 30 per cent. Most cases may be treated expectantly or by phototherapy alone. In one large series, exchange transfusion was needed in only six of 5000 infants of group O mothers. In contrast to rhesus HDNB, the first-born infant is affected in up to 50 per cent of cases. In the rare cases where severe haemolysis occurs, it is likely to be seen again in subsequent pregnancies. The blood film of an infant with ABO-HDNB commonly shows an increase in reticulocytes and spherocytes, but the marked increase in nucleated red cells characteristic of rhesus HDNB is not seen (Table 27.4). The direct antiglobulin test on the infant's blood is often weak or negative, as relatively few antigen-binding sites are present. IgG

Table 27.4
COMPARISON OF FEATURES OF RHESUS (RH) AND ABO INCOMPATIBILITY

	Rh	ABO
First-born affected	Rarely (5 %)	Commonly (50 %)
Severe anaemia	Common	Rare
Stillbirth	Common	Rare
Hepatosplenomegaly	Common	Rare
Direct antiglobulin test (infant)	Positive	Often weak or negative
Spherocytes	Absent	Present
Nucleated red cells	Present	Absent
Exchange transfusion needed	60 %	Less than 1 %

anti-A or anti-B antibodies are usually readily detected in the mother's serum, and a titre of 512 or above is suggestive of haemolytic disease.

COAGULATION DISORDERS IN THE NEWBORN

Evaluation of the coagulation system in the neonate is made difficult by technical factors such as the difficulty in obtaining satisfactory venous blood samples. Capillary blood sampling for coagulation studies is subject to artefact, and samples taken from indwelling catheters are likely to be contaminated with heparin. Microtechniques for blood coagulation studies are available in specialized laboratories. Compared with the older child or adult, the normal neonate has relatively prolonged values for the prothrombin, thrombin and partial thromboplastin times. Levels of the vitamin K-dependent clotting factors and components of the contact pathway (factors XI and XII) are reduced in the normal neonate, whilst factors V and VIII and fibrinogen levels are within normal limits. The bleeding time in the normal neonate is very similar to that of the adult.

Haemorrhagic Disease of the Newborn

Vitamin K-dependent clotting factors (factors II, VII, IX and X) tend to be reduced in the normal neonate because of the absence of vitamin K-producing colonic bacteria and the relative immaturity of hepatocellular synthesis. This combination is exaggerated in the premature infant and, particularly if fed with human breast milk which is relatively poor in vitamin K, such infants may develop a severe haemorrhagic diathesis. Haemorrhagic disease of the newborn was classically seen within three days of birth, but a late form at around 4–6 weeks of age was seen in breast-fed infants. The classical laboratory finding is severe prolongation of the prothrombin time, with lesser elevation of the partial thromboplastin time and normal thrombin time and fibrinogen levels. This disorder is now uncommon in western practice because of the routine administration of water-soluble vitamin K to all premature infants and the fortification of proprietary infant milk formulas.

Disseminated Intravascular Coagulation

Disseminated intravascular coagulation (DIC) is probably more common in the neonatal period than at any other time of life. It is usually seen in the context of a seriously ill, often premature infant with infection, asphyxia, respiratory distress syndrome or necrotizing enterocolitis. Severe thrombocytopenia is common, and typical coagulation changes may be present (see Chapter 13). Serious thrombotic as well as bleeding problems may occur, major vessel thrombosis perhaps being predisposed by the use of central venous or arterial catheters. The treatment of neonatal DIC is essentially that of the underlying cause, although supportive treatment with fresh plasma, cryoprecipitate (as a source of fibrinogen), platelets and possibly heparin may be required.

Inherited Coagulation Disorders

Several inherited coagulation disorders may present in the neonatal period. Bleeding problems in children with classical haemophilia-A or Christmas disease are rare in the first six months of life, but excessive soft tissue bleeding after traumatic 'heel-prick' blood sampling or other manoeuvres may occur. Muscle and joint bleeds start to occur from around six months of age as the child becomes more actively mobile. Deficiency of factor XIII, the fibrin stabilizing factor, may present in the neonatal period with delayed separation and bleeding from the umbilical cord, and a risk of intracerebral haemorrhage is present. Infants homozygous for the recently described vitamin K-dependent anticoagulant factor, protein C, may die in the neonatal period with purpura fulminans.

IRON DEFICIENCY IN CHILDHOOD

Iron is actively transferred from mother to fetus during pregnancy (Chapter 28), the maximal time of transfer being during the third trimester. As a consequence, the premature infant is born with relatively lower iron stores depending on the gestational age. Unless chronic fetomaternal haemorrhage has occurred, iron deficiency anaemia is rare in the first weeks of life. The physiological arrest of erythropoiesis and loss of red cell mass provides a source of re-utilizable iron in the first months of life. However, many infants display iron deficient erythropoiesis between 6–18 months of age, as a period of rapid increase in body mass produces demands on iron in excess of that available from body stores and dietary intake. Iron deficiency is more common in those born prematurely (*see* above) and those in whom weaning on to a mixed diet with a higher iron content is delayed. Cow's milk is relatively poor in iron and, although the concentration of iron in breast milk is similar, it appears to have a much higher bioavailability in the human infant. Proprietary infant feeds are supplemented with iron, as are most cereals. Breast-fed full-term infants do not become iron deficient before six months of age, but those born prematurely need supplements from the second month of life to avoid progressive depletion of iron stores. In the UK, there is a higher incidence of iron deficiency anaemia in children of Asian origin, probably reflecting a lower intake of the highly bioavailable haem iron from meat and the effect of a high phytate intake, e.g. in the form of chapatti flour, which may reduce the absorption of dietary iron. The significance of this so-called 'physiological' iron deficiency of infancy is unclear. There is much evidence of delayed learning ability, irritability and other behavioural or intellectual changes in such children, but interpretation is made difficult by the common association of iron deficiency with socio-economic deprivation and other confounding factors. Evidence of mild iron deficiency may also be seen during the growth spurt of adolescence, especially in menstruating females. All cases of iron deficiency in childhood must be assessed individually and, except in infancy and adolescence, a pathological cause must be strongly considered. Beta-thalassaemia trait must be excluded in children of appropriate ethnic origin with a microcytic blood picture. In the Third World, chronic blood loss from the gastro-intestinal tract due to parasitic disease, especially hook worm, is the commonest cause of iron deficiency anaemia in childhood. In the UK, assessment should include a dietary evaluation and consideration of malabsorption states (in which coexistent folate deficiency would be common), and sources of chronic gastro-intestinal blood loss, such as peptic ulceration and bleeding Meckel's diverticulum, should be considered (Table 27.5). Intolerance of cow's milk may cause occult gastro-intestinal blood loss in infancy as part of an exudative enteropathy, and iron deficiency itself has been associated with an increase in faecal blood loss. Providing that the cause of iron

Table 27.5
CAUSES OF BLOOD LOSS IRON DEFICIENCY ANAEMIA IN CHILDHOOD

Neonate
  Twin-to-twin transfusion
  Fetomaternal haemorrhage
  Bleeding cord
  Venesection for investigation (common in intensive care unit)

Infancy and childhood
  Hiatus hernia
  Cow's milk intolerance
  Gastro-enteritis
  Parasitic infection (e.g. hookworm)
  Meckel's diverticulum
  Peptic ulceration
  Vascular abnormalities
  Menorrhagia in adolescence

deficiency has been determined, treatment with oral iron replacement may be initiated. Ferrous salts are much better absorbed than ferric, and a response rate of approximately 0·3 g/dl of haemoglobin per day may be expected. Liquid preparations are often better tolerated by infants, but older children will usually take ferrous sulphate tablets. Side effects, such as vomiting, abdominal pain and constipation, are generally dose-related and can usually be overcome by a reduction in dosage and administration of iron with food. Failure of an adequate response to oral iron therapy should lead to suspicion of continued blood loss, malabsorption or coexisting inflammatory, malignant or renal disease, although poor compliance is by far the most common problem. Parenteral iron therapy is rarely indicated in childhood, and total dose intravenous infusion of iron dextran carries a risk of anaphylaxis which may be fatal. Sarcoma formation has been reported at the site of intramuscular iron injection.

FURTHER READING

Hinchcliffe R.F., Lilleyman J.S., eds. (1987). *Practical Paediatric Haematology.* Chichester and New York: John Wiley and Sons.

Oski F.A., Naiman J.L. (1982). *Hematologic Problems in the Newborn*, 3rd edn. Philadelphia and London: W.B. Saunders.

Chapter Twenty Eight

Pregnancy and Haematology

INTRODUCTION

In recent decades, improvements in nutrition and standards of antenatal care in developed countries have reduced the incidence of anaemia in pregnancy. However, those of lower socio-economic status, certain ethnic immigrant populations and other defined groups still carry a higher than standard risk. Despite the fall in the incidence of anaemia, haematological problems in pregnancy remain of importance. Thrombo-embolic problems are now a leading cause of maternal death in the UK, and haemorrhage was a major factor in 76 of the 227 deaths attributed directly to pregnancy and childbirth in the UK between 1976 and 1978 (Confidential Enquiry into Maternal Deaths in England and Wales, 1982).

ANAEMIA IN PREGNANCY

Physiological Changes

During normal pregnancy, there is an increase in maternal plasma volume and red cell mass. Little change is seen in the first trimester, but plasma volume then increases by just under 50 per cent by the 35th week of gestation and remains at that level to term. There is a positive correlation between birth weight and plasma volume expansion, and the rise in plasma volume is higher in multiple pregnancies. Maternal red cell mass also increases by an average of 20–30 per cent. However, the relatively greater increase in plasma volume results in a dilutional anaemia and a fall in haematocrit to around 0·3. These changes accommodate the need for increased oxygen transport and the increased volume of circulation in the uteroplacental unit, skin and kidneys. Failure of this physiological plasma expansion in patients with pre-eclamptic toxaemia or hypertension has been linked to suboptimal fetal growth and poorer outcome of pregnancy. There is much current interest in this phenomenon, particularly in relation to changes in whole blood viscosity and flow in the uteroplacental circulation.

Iron Deficiency in Pregnancy

Because of the increased iron demands due to menstruation, a significant proportion of the normal premenopausal female population exists in a state of marginal iron balance, with adequate supplies for normoblastic erythropoiesis but with little or no storage iron. During the course of a normal pregnancy, approximately one gram of extra iron is needed; about 300 mg of this is used to produce fetal red cells and iron stores, and up to 100 mg is present in the feto-placental circulation. In early pregnancy, approximately 500 mg of iron is needed to allow the physiological expansion of maternal red cell mass. These early demands are offset to some extent by the cessation of menstrual loss. In later pregnancy, transfer of iron to the fetus is the major factor. This is an active process and seems to be relatively independent of maternal iron status. By the third trimester, the average iron requirement may reach 6 mg per day, and although the efficiency of iron absorption through the gut may increase up to 50 per cent, the average UK diet contains only about 10 mg of iron per day. Iron deficiency is a virtual certainty in women starting pregnancy with less than 200 mg of storage iron.

The diagnosis of iron deficiency in pregnancy is made more difficult by the physiological fall in haemoglobin and the normal tendency for mean corpuscular volume (MCV) to rise. Serum iron and total iron binding capacity measurements are unreliable in pregnancy, and the best practical parameter of iron stores is the serum ferritin concentration. A serum ferritin level of less than 12 µg/l is indicative of iron deficiency, whereas women with a serum ferritin above 80 µg/l at the booking visit are unlikely to need iron supplements during pregnancy. Although routine iron supplements reliably prevent iron deficiency anaemia in pregnancy, the need for indiscriminant treatment is far from clear. There is no good evidence that subclinical iron deficiency or a mild fall in haemoglobin is detrimental to the outcome of pregnancy, although several studies have shown that significant anaemia results in impaired fetal growth and morbidity. The routine use of iron supplements is also accompanied by poor compliance. In developed countries, providing that the haemoglobin is monitored at regular intervals and those with levels less than 11 g/dl are investigated, prophylactic iron can probably be reserved for the latter part of pregnancy in selected groups, such as those of lower socio-economic status, those with multiple pregnancies and multigravidae.

Megaloblastic Anaemia

Serum levels of vitamin B_{12} fall steadily throughout normal pregnancy due to a combination of haemodilution and active transfer to the fetus. By term, about 30 per cent of women have levels below the normal reference range. However, maternal cobalamin stores are so much greater than the fetal requirement (3000 µg compared with 50 µg) that there is no significant effect on overall cobalamin stores. Indeed, the serum vitamin B_{12} levels rise to normal within a few days of delivery. Pernicious anaemia is rare below 40 years of age, and most women with megaloblastic anaemia of this cause are infertile. Consequently, clinically significant vitamin B_{12} deficiency in pregnancy is an extreme rarity.

On the other hand, folate balance is highly marginal even in developed populations (*see* Chapter 3). The average daily folate requirement in uncomplicated pregnancy is 200–250 µg per day (normal non-pregnant requirement 100 µg). The incidence of clinical folate deficiency tends to reflect the general nutritional status of the population and is much more common in underdeveloped countries, particularly where such diseases as malaria are common. In the UK, megaloblastic anaemia in pregnancy due to folate deficiency is most commonly seen in patients of lower socio-economic status. The incidence is higher in patients with multiple pregnancy and in multigravidae. Most patients with folic acid deficiency are diagnosed late in pregnancy, and an early presentation should raise the suspicion of an underlying factor such as chronic haemolytic anaemia (including sickle-cell disease) or malabsorption. Laboratory diagnosis is hampered by the physiological increase in MCV occurring in normal pregnancy (the MCV may rise by an average of 4 fl, but occasionally up to 20 fl with no evidence of megaloblastic change). Coexisting iron deficiency may also interfere with diagnosis. Serum folate levels are often low in normal pregnancy and although measurement of red cell folate concentration is of more value, this too may be misleadingly normal when folate deficiency occurs rapidly in late pregnancy. Examination of the bone marrow may, however, show marked megaloblastic changes even when the peripheral blood changes are minimal. The routine use of folic acid supplements has not been shown to have a beneficial effect on infant birth weight in well-nourished western populations, and the proposed association between folic acid deficiency and increased incidence of abortion, accidental haemorrhage and toxaemia have not been confirmed. A claim that maternal folate supplementation before conception reduces the frequency of neural tube defects is the subject of a current controlled trial. There is an increasing trend to withhold routine folic acid supplements from patients who belong to well-nourished and low-risk groups and once again to target those patients at particular risk, and this requires the regular haematological evaluation of such patients during the course of the pregnancy.

DISORDERS OF HAEMOGLOBIN IN PREGNANCY

Women with sickle-cell disease (including patients with haemoglobin SC disease and haemoglobin S—β-thalassaemia) have a high incidence of obstetric complications, including pre-eclampsia and thrombotic disease, as well as the usual sickling problems. Maternal morbidity and the spontaneous abortion rate are increased. The infants have a lower than average birth weight and intra-uterine growth retardation is common, possibly due to sickling of red cells in the uteroplacental microcirculation. The value of prophylactic blood transfusion or red cell exchange (to reduce haemoglobin S levels) in pregnancy is controversial. Enthusiasm for this treatment has coincided with improved standards of antenatal, obstetric and neonatal care, and the results of controlled trials are awaited. Folate supplement should be given routinely in view of the high marrow cell turnover. The high morbidity (and mortality) of infants with sickle-cell disease in the first years of life makes it essential for all hospitals to have an appropriate programme of antenatal and neonatal screening for haemoglobinopathies. Prenatal diagnosis of many haemoglobinopathies is now available, and advances in DNA technology have increased the availability of first trimester diagnosis by chorionic villous biopsy, rather than later amniocentesis or fetal blood sampling. Diseases currently identifiable by these techniques include sickle-cell disease and other structural variants such as haemoglobins C and E, many types of β- and α-thalassaemia, and various other disorders such as haemophilia-A or B. Such investigations must be performed in the context of a coordinated programme of screening and counselling.

THROMBOCYTOPENIA IN PREGNANCY

Although a minority of normal patients develop a mild fall in platelet count in late pregnancy, thrombocytopenia is often an indication of significant obstetric complications. Thrombocytopenia may occur in the context of disseminated intravascular coagulation or folic acid deficiency, but immune thrombocytopenia (ITP) is the commonest cause. Women of childbearing age are at highest risk of ITP, and diagnosis is made by the combination of thrombocytopenia despite plentiful marrow megakaryocytes (see Chapter 8). Consistent testing for the presence of platelet antibodies is still only available in a minority of centres. In addition to the risk of maternal haemorrhage, the neonate may be affected by transplacental transmission of IgG platelet antibodies. Historically, the major risk is of neonatal cerebral haemorrhage during vaginal delivery. Conventional management is to give the mother oral steroids if the platelet count falls below $20 \times 10^9/l$ during the course of the pregnancy. Caesarean section may reduce the risk of neonatal haemorrhage. High-dose maternal steroids are often given in late pregnancy, but recent evidence suggests a possible deleterious effect on the neonatal platelet count, possibly by cleaving antibodies from the maternal platelets and freeing them to cross the placenta. High-dose intravenous immunoglobulin administered to the mother in the last 10–14 days of pregnancy may cross the placenta and ameliorate thrombocytopenia in both mother and infant. With this modality, there is an increasing tendency to deliver infants by the vaginal route, and transcervical fetal blood sampling in early labour may be useful in management. Women presenting with ITP in pregnancy should be screened for both systemic lupus erythematosus (also at peak incidence in women of reproductive age) and the lupus anticoagulant (*see* Chapter 23), which is associated with spontaneous abortion and late stillbirths.

COAGULATION DISORDERS IN PREGNANCY

Levels of coagulation factors VII, VIII, X and fibrinogen increase in normal pregnancy and fibrinolytic activity is reduced. The risk of thrombo-embolism is increased, and pulmonary embolism is now the commonest cause of maternal death. Although the highest risk is in the puerperium, about 25 per cent of deaths occur in the antenatal period. Defibrinating and fibrinolytic agents (e.g. ancrod or streptokinase) carry an unacceptable risk of fetal bleeding or placental-site haemorrhage. Warfarin therapy in the first trimester of pregnancy carries a risk of teratogenesis and in late pregnancy may cause fetal haemorrhage. Conventional management of thrombo-embolic disease in pregnancy includes initial full heparinization, switching to warfarin between weeks 12 and 36, and back to heparin until term. Long-term self-administered subcutaneous heparin is an attractive and increasingly used alternative, but it carries a risk of bone demineralization. Anticoagulation is usually continued for six weeks after delivery. Heparin is not effective in women with artificial heart valves and, in this case, the teratogenic risk of warfarin is felt to be exceeded by that of thrombo-embolism. The risk of pulmonary embolism after ceasarean section is up to 16 times that after normal vaginal delivery and recent evidence stresses the safety of low-dose subcutaneous heparin used prophylactically in this setting.

Disseminated intravascular coagulation (DIC) is an accompaniment of many obstetric complications (Table 28.1). DIC is always best controlled by removing the cause which, in pregnancy, commonly means delivery of the fetus or abortus and correction of hypovolaemic or septic shock. Pre-eclampsia is commonly accompanied by platelet consumption, micro-angiopathic haemolysis and changes suggestive of DIC. The cause of pre-eclampsia is poorly understood, but prostacyclin deficiency in the uteroplacental unit may be important. The HELLP syndrome (haemolysis, elevated liver enzymes, low platelets) is

Table 28.1
CAUSES OF DISSEMINATED INTRAVASCULAR COAGULATION IN OBSTETRIC PRACTICE

Abruptio placentae	Hypovolaemic shock
Amniotic fluid embolism	Incompatible blood transfusion
Pre-eclampsia	Fetomaternal haemorrhage
Septic abortion	Septicaemia
Retention of dead fetus	Hypertonic fluids in utero (to induce abortion)

probably a severe variant of pre-eclampsia associated with significant maternal and fetal mortality. The value of prostacyclin infusion is not yet established.

Thrombotic thrombocytopenic purpura and haemolytic uraemic syndrome may be seen in pregnancy. Prostacyclin deficiency may also be important in the aetiology of these disorders, and once a correct diagnosis has been made, management may include infusion of fresh plasma, plasma exchange and prostacyclin infusion.

Pregnancy may be complicated by inherited coagulation disorders. Classical haemophilia is inherited as an X-linked recessive disorder, but occasional female carriers have factor VIII levels low enough to induce excessive puerperal or postoperative bleeding. Autosomal dominant von Willebrand's disease may be the commonest inherited coagulation disorder and is associated with increased risk of postpartum bleeding. Haemorrhage during the pregnancy is rare, perhaps because of the physiological increase in factor VIII and von Willebrand factor. Those with low factor VIII levels at term may be given cryoprecipitate infusion to cover delivery. Operative delivery must be accompanied by careful monitoring of factor levels and replacement therapy.

FURTHER READING

Letsky E.A., ed. (1985). Haematological disorders in pregnancy. *Clinics in Haematology*, **14**(3), 601–805.
Letksy E.A. (1985). *Coagulation Problems During Pregnancy*. Edinburgh and London: Churchill Livingstone.

Chapter Twenty Nine

Old Age and Haematology

It should be stressed that there are no haematological problems specific to old age. Certain diseases such as myelodysplasia and the occurrence of paraproteins are much more common in older people.

This chapter will concentrate on:

1. Anaemia
2. Myeloproliferative disease
3. Malignant disease
4. Paraproteins
5. Coagulation disorders in the elderly.

ANAEMIA

A hypochromic, microcytic anaemia is a common finding, and in the majority of cases, is due to iron deficiency secondary to chronic gastro-intestinal bleeding or, less commonly, poor dietary intake of iron. Serum iron and total iron binding capacity levels should confirm a diagnosis of iron deficiency. A hypochromic, microcytic anaemia may also be present in patients with a chronic disease such as rheumatoid arthritis or other inflammatory or malignant diseases. In this situation, serum iron levels may be low in the absence of iron deficiency and serum ferritin levels are therefore particularly helpful, low levels suggesting iron deficiency. The correct diagnosis of iron deficiency is important, as a chronic lack of iron has deleterious effects on non-haemopoietic tissues. Iron deficiency may reduce cognitive function, work capacity, immunity to infection and alter body temperature regulation.

A macrocytic anaemia may be due to folate deficiency as a result of poor dietary intake. After the patient has been hospitalized, a normal serum folate level may simply reflect an increased folate intake from hospital food, and it may be necessary to perform a red cell folate level which, if reduced, indicates decreased storage of folic acid and, by inference, folic acid deficiency.

When vitamin B_{12} levels are measured 'routinely', a low level in the absence of anaemia or macrocytosis is not infrequently found. Whether serum B_{12} levels fall normally with advancing age remains a controversial point. Many patients with unexpectedly low serum B_{12} levels do not appear to develop any of the haematological manifestations of B_{12} deficiency when observed over many years, and it remains a moot point as to whether such patients should be treated or not.

'True' vitamin B_{12} deficiency is frequently related to pernicious anaemia in the elderly. Previous gastric surgery and blind-loop syndromes are other less common causes. Treatment consists of a series of hydroxycobalamin injections to replenish the stores and, thereafter, life-long treatment by three-monthly injections. In the severely anaemic patient, it is preferable to withhold from giving blood transfusions if possible. Potassium replacement therapy during the early stages of treatment may be desirable, as severe hypokalaemia has been noted in such patients following the commencement of replacement vitamin B_{12} therapy.

MYELOPROLIFERATIVE DISEASES

A raised haemoglobin level is infrequently found in elderly people. Panhyperplasia, splenomegaly and hyperuricaemia point to a diagnosis of polycythaemia vera which, if confirmed, should be treated by either repeated venesections or myelosuppressive therapy to maintain a packed-cell volume (PCV) below 0·45. Secondary polycythaemia may be associated with hypoxia, renal disease or neoplastic disease. The commonest cause of a raised haemoglobin is pseudo- or relative polycythaemia, in which there is no true increase in the circulating red cell mass. The raised haemoglobin value in this situation frequently reflects a lowered plasma volume, which may be secondary to diuretic therapy or gastro-intestinal fluid loss. The measurement of circulating red cell mass and plasma volume is a simple laboratory test which determines whether a patient has true or relative polycythaemia. The treatment of relative polycythaemia is unclear. Whether or not these patients should be venesected to lower their PCV to within the normal range is not known. Our practice is to venesect those patients with a persistent PCV over 0·5 and patients who have a history of thrombotic disease.

MALIGNANT DISEASE

The occurrence and presentation of the myelodysplastic syndromes have been described elsewhere in this book.

Elderly people with acute leukaemia fare badly. It was thought that perhaps they could not tolerate the infectious and bleeding complications associated with chemotherapy. Another reason may be that acute leukaemia in this population is frequently preceded by a myelodysplastic phase, suggesting the presence of disease at a very early stage in the development of haemopoiesis and making the likelihood of eradication of disease by chemotherapy unlikely or very difficult.

Lymphoproliferative diseases tend to have a poor prognosis in elderly people, with the exception perhaps of chronic lymphocytic leukaemia. When Hodgkin's disease occurs, it frequently presents with B-symptoms and advanced stage. Favourable histology is less common, and therefore the prognosis is generally poor. The incidence of non-Hodgkin's lymphoma increases with age. Unfortunately, most patients present with intermediate or high grade histological subtypes. For those patients presenting with low grade lymphomas, the outlook is probably similar to their younger counterparts.

Chemotherapy Tolerance in the Elderly

It has been suggested that elderly people cannot tolerate chemotherapy because either they cannot withstand the complications of treatment or they have less haemopoietic reserve to call on. There is very little concrete evidence to suggest that this is so, with the possible exception of acute leukaemia, where elderly people may have more difficulty in surviving the effects of the prolonged bone marrow hypoplasia which typically follows treatment. Otherwise, the available trials would suggest little, if any, significant differences in drug toxicity when comparing the under 70 and over 70 years age groups. Similarly, the outcome of cancer treatment in terms of response rate and survival is not significantly different in those aged over 70 years compared with their younger counterparts. Perhaps the most important aspect of treating such patients is the presence of concurrent disease of, for example, the heart, liver or kidneys, making patients more vulnerable to the complications of treatment, possibly by altering drug metabolism and excretion rates.

PARAPROTEINS

The presence of a paraprotein in the blood is found in three per cent of people over 70 years of age. The incidence increases with age, and one report suggests a 10 per cent incidence in those over 80 years of age. Using very sensitive techniques, it can be demonstrated that paraproteins may be even more common than that.

The presence of an IgG paraprotein may reflect the presence of a malignant disease, such as multiple myeloma, or may simply be a reflection of a benign event, i.e. benign monoclonal gammopathy (BMG). This is not an accurate title, as long-term follow-up by the Mayo Clinic of patients suspected of having BMG has demonstrated that a significant proportion will further increase their IgG levels or eventually develop a malignant disease, the most common being multiple myeloma. As this may take several years to occur, long-term follow-up of such patients should be considered, and perhaps the term monoclonal gammopathy of undetermined significance (MGUS) is more accurate in these circumstances. The presence of an IgM paraprotein is followed more frequently by a lymphoma such as Waldenström's macroglobulinaemia or amyloidosis.

COAGULATION AND PLATELET DEFECTS

Thrombocytopenia frequently occurs and may be related to drugs such as the thiazide diuretics. Immune thrombocytopenic purpura is less common than in younger patients. Thrombocytopenia, together with neutropenia and/or anaemia, suggests reduced bone marrow activity, and this is frequently secondary to metastatic cancer, myelodysplasia, megaloblastic anaemia, cytotoxic/radiation treatment or alcohol abuse.

Bleeding due to platelet dysfunction may be drug-related, secondary to renal failure or to a bone marrow disease such as myelodysplasia.

Purpura is frequently traumatic in origin. Senile purpura or steroid-induced purpura affects the hands and forearms. Scurvy should be considered in patients living in poor circumstances with typical perifollicular haemorrhages.

FURTHER READING

Hamblin T.J., ed. (1987). Haematological problems in the elderly. *Clinics in Haematology*, 1, 2.

Index

Abetalipoproteinaemia 46
ABO blood group system 127–9
ABO haemolytic disease of
  newborn 242
Acanthocyte 8 (table), 46
Acholuric jaundice 39
Acid citrate dextrose 130
Acid lysis test 46
Activated partial thromboplastin
  time 114
Adriamycin (doxorubicin) 146
Alcohol 225
Allo-immune haemolytic
  anaemia 50
Allopurinol 100
Alveolar macrophages 4
Aminopterin 143
Amyloidosis 178–81
  diagnosis 180–1
  haemodialysis-associated 180
  localized 179 (table), 180
  prognosis 181
  reactive 179, 180 (table)
  senile cardiac 180
  systemic 178–9
  treatment 181
Anaemia
  allo–immune haemolytic 50
  aplastic see aplastic anaemia
  auto-immune haemolytic 47
  chronic disorders
    associated 18, 35–6
  cold antibody auto-immune
    haemolytic 48

congenital Heinz body
  haemolytic 45
Fanconi's 201, 202, 203
haemolytic see haemolytic
  anaemias
iron deficiency see iron
  deficiency anaemia
leuco-erythroblastic 196–7
macrocytic see macrocytic
  anaemia
megaloblastic see megaloblastic
  anaemias
microcytic see microcytic
  anaemia
normochromic 35–6
old people 254–5
pernicious (Addisonian) 31–3
physiological, of infancy 234
pregnancy associated see under
  pregnancy
renal failure associated 228–9
sideroblastic 19–21, 189
  (table), 191 (table)
warm antibody auto-immune
  haemolytic 47–8
Ancrod 217
Anisocytosis 8 (table)
Anticoagulants
  circulating 126
  oral 213–15
Anti-D immunoglobulin 241–2
Antigens
  platelet 129–30
  white cell 129

Antilymphocytic globulin 204–5
Antiplatelet drugs 219–21
Antithrombin III
  concentrate 132 (table)
Antithrombin III deficiency 211
Aplastic anaemia 199–205
  causes 199–201
  complications 203
  hepatitis-induced 222–3
  incidence 201
  investigation 202–3
  pathogenesis 201
  prognosis 203–4
  severe 203 (table)
  symptoms/signs 201–2
  treatment 204–5
Aplastic crises 40
Asparaginase 145
l-asparaginase 210
Aspirin 100, 122, 219, 220–1
Auto-immune haemolytic
  anaemia 47
Auto-immune neutropenia,
  idiopathic 75
Auto-immune
  thrombocytopenia 237

Basophilia 95–6
Basophilic stippling 8 (table)
Basophils 1 (table), 4
Behcet's syndrome 210
Bence–Jones protein 173, 174,
  178, 231
Benign monoclonal
  gammopathy 257
Bernard–Soulier syndrome 116,
  237
Blackfan–Diamond
  syndrome 206
Blackwater fever 52
Bleeding time 113
Blood cells 1 (table)
  measurement 6–7
  production 2–5
Blood formation 2–5
  developmental changes 5

  regulation 5–6
Blood groups 127
Blood transfusion
  complications 127–37,
    133–7
  air embolism 135
  allergic reactions 134
  circulatory overload 135
  haemolytic transfusion
    reactions 133–4
  infection transmission 134–5
  iron overload 136
  massive transfusion 124, 135–6
  purpura 136–7
Plasma components 131, 132–3
  (table)
  concentrated (packed) 130
  platelet concentrates 131
  red cells 130–1
  white cell-depleted blood 131
B-lymphocytes 1 (table), 4
Bone marrow 5
Burr cell 8 (table)
Busulphan 100, 154, 186

Carpal tunnel syndrome 180
Chapatti flour 245
Childhood
  blood count changes 234–5
  idiopathic thrombocytopenic
    purpura 237–8
  iron deficiency 244–6
  'physiological' 245
  see also neonate
Chlorambucil 158, 186
Christmas disease 116–20
Citrate phosphate plus
  adenine 130
Clostridium welchii exotoxin 51
Coagulation cascade 110 (fig),
  111–12
Coeliac disease 165
Coagulation disorders
  liver disease 123–4, 223–7
  neonatal 243–4
  pregnant women 252–3

Index

Coagulation factor assays 114
Coagulation factor
 disorders 116–22
Coagulation function tests 114
Cold agglutinin disease,
 secondary 49
Cold antibody auto-immune
 haemolytic anaemia 48
Cold haemagglutinin disease
 (CHAD) 48 (table), 49
Collagen diseases 19
Congenital Heinz-body
 haemolytic anaemia 45
Corticosteroids (steroids) 146,
 147, 158, 238
Cryoprecipitate 132 (table)
Cyclic neutropenia 76
Cyclo-oxygenase deficiency 116
Cyclophosphamide 146
Cytosine arabinoside 146, 192

DAT (6-thioguanine) 146
Duanorubicin 145
Deamino-8-D-arginine
 vasopressin 119–20
Deoxycoformycin 161
1,25-dihydroxy vitamin D_3 192
Diamond–Blackfan
 syndrome 206
Dipyridamole 219, 220
Discocyte 8 (table)
Disseminated intravascular
 coagulation 80, 125
 neonatal 244
 obstetric complication 252
Donath–Landsteiner antibody 49
Doxorubicin (Adriamycin) 146
Drugs
 immune haemolytic
  anaemia-inducing 50–1
 'innocent bystander'
  phenomenon 50–1
 neutropenia-inducing 74, 75
  (table)
 platelet dysfunction
  inducing 122

Dyserythropoiesis 46–7
Dysfibrinogenaemia 211
 (table), 212

Elderly see Old age
Electronic cell counters 7 (table)
Elliptocyte 8 (table)
Elliptocytosis, hereditary 42
Embden-Meyerhof pathway 37
Eosinophilia 22–4
Eosinophils 1 (table), 3
Erythroblastosis foetalis 239
Erythrocytes see red blood cells
Erythrocytosis see polycythaemia
Erythropoietin 5, 228, 229
Evan's syndrome 82

Factor II concentrate 132 (table)
Factor VII concentrate 132
 (table)
Factor VIII concentrate 132
 (table)
Factor VIII inhibitor bypassing
 activity 120
Factor IX concentrate 132
 (table)
Factor X concentrate 132 (table)
Familial Mediterranean
 fever 179, 181
Fanconi's syndrome 201, 202,
 203
Felty's syndrome 75–6
Ferrous fumarate 17
Ferrous sulphate 17
Fibrin degradation products 112
Fibrinolysis 112, 113 (fig)
Fibrinolytic activity tests 114–15
Fibrinolytic agents 217–18
Folates 25–6
Folic acid 21
Folic acid deficiency 25–8
 causes 27 (table)
 clinical features 27–8
 diagnosis 28
 treatment 33
Fresh frozen plasma 132 (table)

Gaisböck's syndrome
    (spurious/relative/stress
    polycythaemia) 182, 184
Glanzmann's
    thrombasthenia 116
Glycolytic pathway 42–3
Glucose-6-phosphate
    dehydrogenase
    deficiency 43–4
    drugs causing haemolysis 44
        (table)
Granulocytes 1 (table), 3–4

Haematocrit 7 (table)
Haem molecules 53
Haemoglobin
    catabolism 40 (fig)
    disorders 44–6
    fetal, hereditary persistence 53
    low affinity 73
    measurement 7 (table)
    structural variants 54 (table)
    unstable 71
Haemoglobin A 59
Haemoglobin Barts 59
Haemoglobin Bristol 45
Haemoglobin C 45, 71 (fig)
Haemoglobin Chesapeake 45
Haemoglobin D 71 (table)
Haemoglobin E 45, 71 (table)
Haemoglobin F 5, 59
Haemoglobin H 59
Haemoglobin H disease 59
Haemoglobin Hammersmith 45
Haemoglobin Köln 45
Haemoglobin Lepore 57, 58
    (table)
Haemoglobin Ms 45, 72
Haemoglobin S 45, 63, 65 (fig)
Haemoglobin SC disease 45
Haemoglobinopathies 53–73
    classification 53 (table)
    geography 55
    high affinity 72
    incidence 55
    inheritance 54

prenatal diagnosis 251
Haemolysis 37–40
    chronic liver disease 52
    chronic renal failure 52
    drug-induced 50 (table)
    intravascular 39
    micro-angiopathic 51
    'toxic' 51–2
Haemolytic anaemias 37–52
    acquired 46–52
    classification 38–9 (table)
    complications 40–1
    drug-induced immune 50–1
Haemolytic transfusion
    reactions 133–4
Haemolytic uraemic
    syndrome 230–1, 253
Haemophilia 116–20
    female carriers 253
Haemopoiesis regulation 5–6
Haemostasis 110–12
    congenital disorders 115–22
Ham's test 46
Hand-foot syndrome 66
Heinz bodies 8 (table), 45
HELLP syndrome 252–3
Heparin 210, 215–17
Hepatitis 222–3
    chronic active 223
Hereditary elliptocytosis 42
Hereditary spherocytosis 41–2
High affinity
    haemoglobinopathies 72
Histiocytes (macrophages) 1
    (table), 4
Hodgkin's disease 168–71
    background 168
    classification 169 (table)
    complications 170
    differential diagnosis 170
    investigation 169
    old people 256
    pathology 168
    prognosis 171
    symptoms/signs 168–9
    treatment 170

Homozygous haemoglobin C
    disease 71
Howell-Jolly bodies 8 (table)
Human albumin solutions 132
    (table)
Hydrops foetalis 59
Hydroxyurea 100, 186, 187
Hydroxycobalamin 33–4
Hypercoagulability 207
Hypereosinophilic sydrome 93–4
Hypersplenism 80, 87, 107–8,
    226 (table)
Hyperviscosity syndrome 175,
    210
Hyposplenism 108–9
Idiopathic auto-immune
    neutropenia 75
Immunoglobulins 172–3
    fractions 132 (table)
'Innocent bystander'
    phenomenon 50–1
α-interferon 100, 154, 161
Intravenous immunoglobulin
    (IVIG) therapy 236, 237,
    238, 251
Iron
    daily requirements 12 (table)
    deficiency 12
        'physiological' in
            childhood 245
        pregnancy 148–9
        sarcoma at intramuscular
            injection site 246
Iron deficiency anaemia 11–18
    aetiology 11
    childhood 244–6
    complications 16–17
    differential diagnosis 15–16
    geography 12
    incidence 12
    investigations 14–15
    prevention 17
    symptoms/signs 13
    treatment 17–18
Iron edetate 17
Iso-immune neutropenia 75

Iso-immune
    thrombocytopenia 236–7
Jaundice, obstructive 223, 226
Kaolin cephalin clotting
    time 114, 115 (table)
Koilonychia 13
Kupffer cells 4
Leptocyte (target cell) 8 (table)
Leucocytes *see* white blood cells
Leucocytosis 90–6
Leucoencephalopathy 145
Leuco-erythroblastic
    anaemia 196–7
Leukaemia, acute 138–50
    aetiology 138–9
    bone marrow
        transplantation 147–50
        autologous 149
        compatible sibling 148–9
        HLA-matched unrelated
            donor 149
        mismatched 149
    classification 141–2
    complications 147
    differential diagnosis 143
    incidence 139
    investigations 140–1
    pathology 139
    prognosis 150
    symptoms/signs 139–40
    treatment 143–7
Leukaemia, acute
    lymphoblastic 139
    classification 141 (table), 142
        (table)
    prognosis 150
    treatment 144–50
Leukaemia, acute myeloid 139
    classification 141 (table)
    prognosis 150
    treatment 146–7
Leukaemia, chronic
    lymphocytic 155–9
    aetiology 155

Leukaemia, chronic – *continued*
  complications 157
  investigations 156
  pathology 155
  prognosis 159
  staging 157 (table)
  symptoms/signs 156
  treatment 158
Leukaemia, chronic
    myeloid 151–5
  aetiology 151
  complications 153–4
  investigations 153
  pathology 151–2
  prognosis 155
  symptoms/signs 153
  treatment 154
Leukaemia, chronic
    myelomonocytic 189
Leukaemia, eosinophilic 94
Leukaemia, hairy-cell (leukaemic
    reticulo-endotheliosis) 159–<
  aetiology 159
  complications 161
  differential diagnosis 160–1
  investigations 160
  pathology 160
  prognosis 162
  symptoms/signs 160
  treatment 161
Leukaemia, monocytic 147
Leukaemia, prolymphocytic 159
Leukaemia, promyelocytic 142
Leukaemia, secondary 193–4
Liver
  biopsy, prothrombin time 227
  chronic failure 223–4
  cirrhosis 223–4
  disorders 52, 123–4, 222–7
Loeffler's pneumonia
    (syndrome) 93
Low affinity haemoglobins 73
Lupus anticoagulant 126, 209
Lymphocytes 1 (table)
  B- 1 (table), 4

  T- 1 (table), 4–5
Lymphocytosis 94–5
Lymphoma
  cutaneous 165, 167–8
  non-Hodgkin's *see*
    non-Hodgkin's lymphoma

Macrocytic anaemia 23–24
  treatment 33–4
Macrocytosis 8 (table), 23
  causes 23 (table)
  differential diagnosis 24
Macrophages (histiocytes) 1
    (table), 4
Malaria 51–2
Malignant disease 256
Malignant myelosclerosis (acute
    myelofibrosis) 198
M-AMSA 146
Marrow failure, single cell
    lines 205–6
Massive transfusion
    syndrome 124, 135–6
May-Hegglin syndrome 237
Mean corpuscular haemoglobin
    (MCH) 6 (table), 7
    (table)
Mean corpuscular haemoglobin
    concentration (MCHC) 6
    (table)
Mean corpuscular volume
    (MCV) 6 (table), 7
    (table)
Mean platelet volume 7 (table)
Megakaryocytes 4
Megaloblastic anaemias 24–5
  in pregnancy 249–50
  treatment 33–4
6-mercaptopurine 145
Methotrexate 145
Micro-angiopathic haemolysis 51
Microcytic anaemia 10–22
  causes 10 (table)
  chronic disorders 18
  investigations 16 (table)

Index 265

Microcytosis 8 (table)
Mitozantrone 147
Monoclonal gammopathy of undetermined significance 173–4
Monocytes 1 (table), 4
Monocytosis 95
M-proteins (paraproteins) 172–3, 257
Multiple myeloma 231–2
Mycosis fungoides (Sézary's syndrome) 164 (table), 165
Myelodysplasia 188–94
  classification 189 (table)
  primary 188–92
    background 188
    complications 190–1
    differential diagnosis 190
    pathology 188
    prognosis 192
    treatment 191–2
  prognosis 189 (table)
  secondary 193–4
Myelofibrosis 195–8
  acute (malignant myelosclerosis) 198
  primary 195–8
    background 196
    investigation 196–7
    pathology 196
    prognosis 198
    symptoms/signs 196
    treatment 197
Myeloid leukaemoid reaction 90–1
Myelomatosis 174–6
  diagnosis 174
  investigations 175
  prognosis 175–6
  symptoms/signs 174–6
  treatment 175–6
Myeloproliferative syndromes 208–9
  old people 255–6

Neonate
  ABO haemolytic disease 242–3
  blood 234–5
  coagulation disorders 243–4
    inherited 244
  disseminated intravascular coagulation 244
  haemolytic disease 238–9
  Rhesus haemolytic disease 239–42
  thrombocytopenia 235–7
Nephrotic syndrome 210
Neutropenia 74–7
  cyclic 76
  idiopathic auto-immune 75
  immune-mediated 75–6
  infection-induced 75
  investigation 77
  iso-immune 75
  racial incidence 74
  systemic lupus erythematosus associated 76
Neutrophilia 90–1
Neutrophil polymorphs 1 (table), 3
Non-Hodgkin's lymphomas 162–8
  background 163
  classification 164 (table)
  complications 166
  cutaneous 165, 167–8
  differential diagnosis 166
  high grade 164 (table), 167
  intermediate grade 164 (table), 167
  investigations 166
  low grade 164 (table), 167
  pathology 163–4
  prognosis 166–8
  staging system 165 (table)
  symptoms/signs 164–5
  treatment 166–8
Normochromic anaemias 35–6

Obstructive jaundice 223, 226

Old age 254-8
  anaemia 254-5
  chemotherapy tolerance 256-7
  coagulation defects 257-8
  immune thrombocytopenic
    purpura 257
  malignant disease 256
  myeloproliferative
    diseases 255-6
  paraproteins 257
  platelet defects 257-8
Osteoclast activating factor 175
Oxygen transport
    abnormalities 54

Packed-cell volume 7
Paediatric haematology 234-46
Pancytopenia 87-9
Pappenheimer's bodies 8 (table)
Paraproteins (M-proteins) 172-3, 257
Paroxysmal cold
  haemoglobinuria 49-50
Paroxysmal nocturnal
  haemoglobinuria 45-7, 201
Paterson-Kelly syndrome
  (Plummer-Vinson
  syndrome) 13
Pelger-Hüet abnormality 189
Pernicious anaemia
  (Addisonian) 31-3
Phenindione 213
Physiological anaemia of
  infancy 234
PIVKA (protein induced by
  vitamin K absence) 226
Plasmin 112
Plasminogen 112
Plasminogen activator
  deficiency 211 (table)
Plateletcrit 7
Platelets 1 (table), 4
  activity tests 112-13
  antigens 129-30

concentrates 131
count 7 (table), 112
infancy/childhood 235
disorders 115-16
dysfunction 113
  drug-induced 122
  renal disease 229-30
  systemic diseases 122-3
enzyme deficiencies 116
intracellular defects 116
in vitro aggregation 113
membrane abnormalities 116
prostaglandin metabolism 117
  (fig)
Plummer-Vinson syndrome
  (Paterson-Kelly
  syndrome) 13
Poikilocytosis 8 (table)
Polycythaemia
  (erythrocytosis) 182-7
  primary 185
  prognosis 187
  relative (spurious/stress
    polycythaemia; Gaisböck's
    syndrome) 182, 184
  management 187
  renal disease associated 230
  secondary 183 (table), 184, 185
  management 187
Polycythaemia vera 182-3
  management 186
  old people 255
  thrombosis 208-9
Portal hypertension 223
Prednisolone 144, 238
Pre-eclampsia 252-3
Pregnancy 247-53
  anaemia 247-50
    megaloblastic 249-50
  coagulation disorders 252-3
  disseminated intravascular
    coagulation 252
  haemoglobin disorders 250-1
  HELLP syndrome 252-3

iron deficiency 248-9
physiological changes 247-8
thrombocytopenia 251-2
thrombotic thrombocytopenic purpura 253
Prostacyclin 219, 220-1
Protein C deficiency 211
Protein induced by vitamin K absence (PIVKA) 226
Protein S deficiency 211
Prothrombin time 114, 115 (table)
Pure red cell aplasia 205-6
Purpura
  acute thrombocytopenic 82
  chronic idiopathic thrombocytopenic 78-9, 82
    investigation 82-3
    treatment 84-6
  idiopathic thrombocytopenic, in childhood 237-8
  immune thrombocytopenic 257
  senile 258
  steroid-induced 258
  thrombotic thrombocytopenic 230-1
  traumatic 258
Pyridoxine 21
Pyruvate kinase deficiency 43

Radiation somnolence syndrome 145
Radiophosphorous 100, 186
Recombinant granulocyte-monocyte colony stimulating factor (GM-CSF) 6
Red blood cells (erythrocytes) 1 (table, 2-3)
  basophilic stippling 8 (table)
  count 7 (table)
  fragmentation 8 (table), 51
  inclusion bodies 8 (table)
  morphology 8 (table)
  neonatal 235
  pure aplasia 205-6
Renal disease 228-32
  anaemia associated 228-9
  haemostatic defects 229-30
  multiple myeloma associated 231-2
  polycythaemia associated 230
  sickle-cell disease associated 232
Renal failure, chronic 52
Renal transplantation 232
Reticulocytes 2-3
Reticulo-endothelial blockade 19
13-*cis* retinoic acid 192
Rhesus anti-D immunoglobulin 241-2
Rhesus blood group system 129
Rhesus haemolytic disease of newborn 239-42
Rheumatoid arthritis 19
Richter's syndrome 157

Sarcoma, at intramuscular iron injection site 246
Scurvy 258
Sézary's syndrome (mycosis fungoides) 164 (table), 165
Sickle C disease 69-70
Sickle-cell (drepanocyte) 8 (table)
Sickle-cell disease 44, 64-9
  clinical presentation 64-7
  crisis 65-6
    aplastic 66-7
    haemolytic 66 (table), 67
    infarctive (painful) 65-6
    sequestration 66
  investigation 67-8
  pregnant women 250
  prognosis 68
  renal disease associated 232
  treatment 68-9

Sickle-cell trait 63–4
Sickle β-thalassaemia 70–1
Sickling disorders 63–71
Sideroblastic anaemias 19–21,
    189 (table), 191 (table)
Solitary plasmacytoma of
    bone 174
Spherocyte 8 (table)
Spherocytosis, hereditary 41–2
Splenectomy 106–7
Splenomegaly 102–7
    aetiology 102–4
    investigation 105–6
    symptoms/signs 104–5
    treatment 106–7
Steroids (corticosteroids) 146,
    147, 158, 238
Stomatocyte 8 (table)
Streptokinase 217–18
Sulphinpyrazone 219–20, 220
Systemic lupus erythematosus 76,
    209
    pancytopenia 87
    platelet antibodies 79
    thrombocytopenic purpura
        associated 84

Target cell (leptocyte) 8 (table)
TAR (thrombocytopenia-absent
    radius) syndrome 237
Thalassaemia 45–6, 55–63
    alpha-(α-) 22
        clinical presentation 59–60
        genetics 57
        geographical distribution 56
            (tables)
        incidence 55
        investigation 59–60
        silent 60
        trait 59
    antenatal diagnosis 62–3
    beta-(β-) 21
        clinical presentation 60–1
        genetics 57
        investigation 60–1

    sickle 70–1
    family studies 61
    geography 55–7
    incidence 55
    intermedia 58 (table), 61
    major 58 (table), 61
    minor 61
    molecular basis 59
    pathology 57
    prevention 62
    structural haemoglobinopathies
        interaction 58 (table)
    treatment 61–2
6-thioguanine (DAT) 146
Thrombasthenia,
    Glanzmann's 116
Thrombin time 114, 115 (table)
Thrombocythaemia, primary 97,
    98
    differential diagnosis 99
    investigation 99
    prognosis 100
    thrombosis 208–9
    treatment 99–100
Thrombocytopenia 78–86
    aetiology 78–80
    auto-immune 236
    differential diagnosis 83–4
    incidence 80
    investigation 82–3
    iso-immune 236–7
    neonatal 235–7
    old people 257–8
    pregnant women 251–2
    prognosis 86
    symptoms/signs 80–1
Thrombocytopenia-absent radius
    (TAR) syndrome 237
Thrombocytosis 97–100
    causes 98 (table)
    differential diagnosis 99
    investigation 99
    pathology 97
    prognosis 100
    symptoms/signs 97–8

transient 99
treatment 99–100
Thrombopoietin 5–6
Thrombosis 207–12
  primary causes 210–12
  secondary causes 208–10
Thrombotic thrombocytopenic
  purpura 230–1, 253
Thromboxane synthetase
  deficiency 116
Ticlopidine 220
Tissue plasminogen activator 218
Tissue plasminogen activator
  inhibitor 211
T-lymphocytes 1 (table), 4–5
TORCH 81
Trousseau's syndrome 209
Tuberculosis 19
Tumour lysis syndrome 166

Unstable haemoglobins 71
Urokinase 217–18

Vincristine 144
Virchow's triad 207

Vitamin B_{12} deficiency 28–30
  causes 29–30
  investigations 32–3
  treatment 33–4
Vitamin K 112, 226
  deficiency 124, 226
Von Willebrand's disease 120–2
  pregnant women 253
Von Willebrand factor (factor
  VIII) 112, 120, 253
VP-16 145–6, 146

Waldenström's
  macroglobulinaemia 177–8
Warfarin 213–15, 220
  in pregnancy 215
Warm antibody auto-immune
  haemolytic anaemia 47–8
White blood cells (leucocytes) 1
  (table), 3–5
  antigens 129
  count 7 (table)
Wiskott-Aldrich syndrome 237
Wound Infection 19